Emerging Pandemics

Pandemics are often associated with viruses and bacteria occurring in wildlife in natural environments. Thus, diseases of epidemic and pandemic scale are mostly zoonotic, some of which include AIDS, Zika virus, severe acute respiratory syndrome (SARS), and COVID-19. The book seeks to explore the documented history of pandemics and various epidemics that have the potential of turning into pandemics with the warming climate, pollution, and environmental destruction.

The book covers some of the most essential elements of the diseases of pandemic nature and their relationship with the environment:

- Environment as a reservoir of human diseases
- Climate change: emerging driver of infectious diseases
- Occurrence and environmental dimensions of specific pandemics and epidemics
- Pandemics, environment, and globalisation: understanding the interlinkage in the context of COVID-19
- Climate change and zoonotic diseases: malaria, plague, dengue, encephalitis
- Tuberculosis: an old enemy of mankind and possible next pandemic
- Lassa fever in Nigeria: case fatality ratio, social consequences, and prevention

There are cases where scientists fear that many epidemics have the potential of turning into pandemics, if we do not pay attention to them, and measures are not being taken to control these occurrences. This book attempts to provide integrated risk assessment on pandemics like COVID-19. It covers fundamental factors of global disease outbreaks through the complexity and severity of consequences. The information collated in this book will help in the design of mitigation measures, including behavioural changes that could prevent the emergence of such pandemics, thus protecting human life and minimising losses incurred due to diseases of such magnitude.

Emerging Pandemics

Connections with Environment and Climate Change

Edited by
Sadaf Nazneen, Akebe Luther King Abia, and Sughosh Madhav

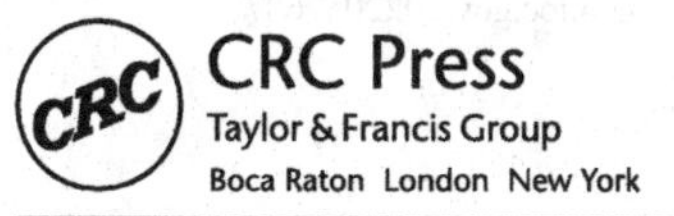

CRC Press is an imprint of the
Taylor & Francis Group, an informa business

First edition published 2023
by CRC Press
6000 Broken Sound Parkway NW, Suite 300, Boca Raton, FL 33487-2742

and by CRC Press
2 Park Square, Milton Park, Abingdon, Oxon, OX14 4RN

CRC Press is an imprint of Taylor & Francis Group, LLC

Library of Congress Cataloging-in-Publication Data

Names: Nazneen, Sadaf, editor. | Abia, Akebe Luther King, editor. | Madhav, Sughosh, editor.
Title: Emerging pandemics : connections with environment and climate change / edited by Sadaf Nazneen, Akebe Luther King Abia, Sughosh Madhav.
Description: Boca Raton : CRC Press, 2022. | Includes bibliographical references and index.
Identifiers: LCCN 2022059686 (print) | LCCN 2022059687 (ebook) | ISBN 9781032265346 (hardback) | ISBN 9781032265353 (paperback) | ISBN 9781003288732 (ebook)
Subjects: LCSH: Epidemics--Environmental aspects. | Pandemics--Environmental aspects. | Environmental degradation--Health aspects.
Classification: LCC RA652 .E445 2022 (print) | LCC RA652 (ebook) | DDC 614.4/9--dc23/eng/20230420
LC record available at https://lccn.loc.gov/2022059686
LC ebook record available at https://lccn.loc.gov/2022059687

ISBN: 978-1-032-26534-6 (hbk)
ISBN: 978-1-032-26535-3 (pbk)
ISBN: 978-1-003-28873-2 (ebk)

DOI: 10.1201/9781003288732

Typeset in Times
by Deanta Global Publishing Services, Chennai, India

Contents

Preface vii
Editor Biographies ix
Contributors xi

Chapter 1 Occurrence and Environmental Dimensions of Specific Pandemics and Epidemics 1

Juliet Adamma Shenge

Chapter 2 Climate Change: Emerging Driver of Infectious Diseases 17

Ayukafangha Etando and Akebe Luther King Abia

Chapter 3 Economic Outcomes of Emerging Pandemics and Their Implications for the Environment 33

Denis Nfor Yuni and Lehlohonolo Mantsi

Chapter 4 Tuberculosis: An Old Enemy of Mankind and Possible Next Pandemic 47

Chitra Rani, Raj Kishor Pandey, and Shah Ubaid-ullah

Chapter 5 Pandemics, Environment, and Globalisation: Understanding the Interlinkage in the Context of COVID-19 63

Mantosh Kumar Satapathy, Hemant Kumar, Chih-Hao Yang, Ting-Lin Yen, and Papita Das

Chapter 6 Climate Change and Zoonotic Diseases: Malaria, Plague, Dengue, and Encephalitis 81

Raj Kishor Pandey, Amit Kumar Dubey, Simran Sharma, and Chitra Rani

Chapter 7 Environmental Dimensions of Zika Virus Triggered Outbreak and Its Association with Neurological Complications Like Guillain–Barré Syndrome and Microcephaly 99

Ishfaq Ahmad Ahanger and Shah Ubaid-ullah

Chapter 8 Emerging Contaminants in the Environment and Their Linkage with COVID-19 117

Majid Peyravi and Marjan Sadat Mirmasoomi

Chapter 9 Lassa Fever in Nigeria: Case Fatality Ratio, Social Consequences, and Prevention 133

Sylvester Chibueze Izah, Adams Ovie Iyiola, Wisdom Richard Poyeri, and Kurotimipa Frank Ovuru

Chapter 10 Contribution of Anthropogenic Factors to the Global Advancement of Zika Virus 151

Manika Vij, Sai Aditya Reddy Lingampally, and Saurabh Pande

Index 167

Preface

Despite technological advances that have facilitated disease diagnosis and improved treatment, humanity continues to suffer from numerous epidemics and pandemics. While some of these pandemics are recent, like COVID-19, some of them were once forgotten and have resurfaced unexpectedly. The emergence of these new pandemics and the re-emergence of some forgotten ones are largely influenced by human activities in the environment. Despite this realisation, interventions to curb these diseases focus on humans and animals, with little attention given to the environment. However, it is well established today that the environment plays a crucial role in disease reservoirs and sources. Therefore, it is also widely acknowledged that a critical understanding of the environmental dimension of most human diseases is vital for fighting disease outbreaks and spread. The world is now gradually emerging from the mayhem of COVID-19, and now is the time to take a holistic overview of the situation to avoid pandemics of this magnitude in future. Unsustainable human activities, loss of wildlife habitat, and warming climate may trigger many such events in the future. The idea of compiling a book wherein the role of environment and climate is discussed emerged from the fact that most of the diseases of epidemic and pandemic nature are zoonotic in nature, with environment as their reservoir. The book encompasses the role of environment and climate change in the outbreak of these diseases, their impact on environment, society, and economy, and methods of surveillance.

The book *Emerging Pandemics: Connections with Environment and Climate Change* presents an in-depth review of the current state of human pandemics and their relation to the environment in ten chapters from across the globe. The book opens with specific pandemics and their link to the environment. Three chapters address how climate change influences the occurrence of pandemics. Three other chapters point to viral disease outbreaks such as Zika and Lassa fever, their association with anthropogenic activities, and their socio-economic implications. The re-emergence of old diseases like tuberculosis and their pandemic potential is elucidated in another chapter. Finally, the environmental dimension of COVID-19 and its association with emerging contaminants are elaborated. Finally, focusing on COVID-19, one chapter looks at the link between pandemics, the environment, and globalisation.

This book is a valuable masterpiece, serving as a reference book for the research community working with pandemics, and researchers and scholars looking at understanding the contribution of the environment to disease spread. It may also be used as a textbook for graduate-level epidemiology and public health courses.

Editor Biographies

SADAF NAZNEEN

Dr Sadaf Nazneen has a PhD in Environmental Sciences from the School of Environmental Sciences, Jawaharlal Nehru University, New Delhi, India. She works on the interface of Environmental Chemistry and Biology. Dr Nazneen has over 10 years of experience in various fields related to environmental pollution, nutrient cycling, carbon sequestration, and climate change. Dr Nazneen has an MSc degree in Biosciences and has sound knowledge of biological and environmental subjects. Currently, she is Dr D. S. Kothari Postdoctoral Fellow in the Department of Civil Engineering, Jamia Millia Islamia, New Delhi, India. Her area of research is Coastal Biogeochemistry and Ecology. For her PhD, she worked on Chilika Lagoon, Asia's largest lagoon and a Ramsar Site. She has published several papers, book chapters, and conference papers out of her PhD work. She is also actively involved in teaching Civil and Environmental Engineering students in her department.

AKEBE LUTHER KING ABIA

Akebe Luther King Abia (King) is a Professor of Applied and Environmental Microbiology at the University of KwaZulu-Natal. He is also the founder and chief executive officer of the Environmental Research Foundation. His research focuses on, but is not limited to, antimicrobial resistance in the environment and how this relates to humans and animals through the One Health approach, using culture and molecular techniques, including metagenomics and whole-genome sequencing. He has over 20 years of experience as a microbiologist and is involved in many projects, including monitoring water and soil for human pathogens, especially antibiotic-resistant ones, under changing climates. He has published over 80 journal articles, 6 chapters, and 1 book. He has also graduated several PhD and MSc students.

SUGHOSH MADHAV

Dr Sughosh Madhav is presently working as Dr D. S. Kothari Postdoctoral Fellow in the Department of Civil Engineering, Jamia Millia Islamia, New Delhi, India. He obtained his master's degree from the Department of Environmental Science, Banaras Hindu University, Varanasi, India. He earned his doctorate from Jawaharlal Nehru University, New Delhi. The area of his doctoral research is the environmental impact of industrial effluents on groundwater and soil quality. He has published various research papers and book chapters in the field of environmental geochemistry, water pollution, wastewater remediation, and climate change. He has also edited seven books in Wiley, Springer, and Elsevier publications on various environmental issues.

Contributors

Akebe Luther King Abia
Antimicrobial Research Unit
College of Health Sciences
University of Kwazulu-Natal
Durban, South Africa

Ishfaq Ahmad Ahanger
Centre for Interdisciplinary Research in Basic Sciences
Jamia Millia Islamia
Jamia Nagar
New Delhi, India

Papita Das
Department of Chemical Engineering
Jadavpur University
Kolkata 700032, India

Amit Kumar Dubey
Department of Biotechnology
National Institute of Pharmaceutical Education and Research
Hajipur, India

Ayukafangha Etando
Department of Medical Laboratory Sciences
Faculty of Health Sciences
Eswatini Medical Christian University
Mbabane, Eswatini

Adams Ovie Iyiola
Department of Fisheries and Aquatic Resources Management
Faculty of Renewable Natural Resources Management
Osun State University
Osogbo, Nigeria

Sylvester Chibueze Izah
Department of Microbiology
Faculty of Science
Bayelsa Medical University
Yenagoa, Bayelsa State, Nigeria

Hemant Kumar
Dr. B. R. Ambedkar National Institute of Technology
Jalandhar, Punjab 144027, India

Sai Aditya Reddy Lingampally
Department of Material Sciences and Convergence Technology
Gyeongsang National University
Jinju Si, South Korea

Lehlohonolo Mantsi
Department of Economics
National University of Lesotho
Roma, Lesotho

Marjan Sadat Mirmasoomi
Nanotechnology Research Institute
Babol Noshirvani University of Technology
Babol, Iran

Kurotimipa Frank Ovuru
Neglected Tropical Diseases Programme
Directorate of Public Health
Ministry of Health Bayelsa State Nigeria
Yenagoa, Nigeria

Raj Kishor Pandey
Post-Doctoral Department of Child Health
School of Medicine
University of Missouri-Columbia
Columbia, MO

Saurabh Pandey
Magstik Pvt. Ltd.
Puresaun, Sultanpur, India

Majid Peyravi
Department of Chemical Engineering
Babol Noshirvani University of Technology
Babol, Iran

Wisdom Richard Poyeri
Directorate of Nursing Services
Ministry of Health Bayelsa State Nigeria
Yenagoa, Nigeria

Chitra Rani
University of Connecticut Health Center
Farmington, CT, USA

Mantosh Kumar Satapathy
Department of Pharmacology
School of Medicine
College of Medicine
Taipei Medical University
No. 250, Wuxing St., Taipei 110, Taiwan

Simran Sharma
Department of Basic and Applied Sciences
National Institute of Food Technology and Entrepreneurship & Management
Kundli, Sonepat, Haryana, India

Juliet Adamma Shenge
Virology Research Unit
Department of Biological Sciences
Dominican University
Ibadan, Nigeria

Shah Ubaid-ullah
J&K Higher Education Department
Department of Biotechnology
Islamia College of Science and Commerce
Srinagar, Jammu and Kashmir, India

Manika Vij
Department of Dermatology
Medical Faculty
Medical Center
University of Freiburg
Freiburg im Breisgau, Germany

Chih-Hao Yang
Department of Pharmacology
School of Medicine
College of Medicine
Neuroscience Research Center
Taipei Medical University
Taipei 110, Taiwan

Ting-Lin Yen
Department of Medical Research
Cathay General Hospital
Taipei 22174, Taiwan

Denis Nfor Yuni
Department of Economics
National University of Lesotho
Roma, Lesotho

1 Occurrence and Environmental Dimensions of Specific Pandemics and Epidemics

Juliet Adamma Shenge

CONTENTS

1.1 Introduction 1
1.2 Global Trend of Viral Disease Outbreaks 3
1.3 Human Immunodeficiency Virus (HIV)/Acquired Immunodeficiency Syndrome (AIDS) 3
1.4 HIV/AIDS Epidemiology and Impacts in Africa 4
1.5 Relationship Between HIV/AIDS and the Environment 5
1.6 Ebola Viral Disease Outbreak and Re-emergence 6
1.7 Environmental Impact of Ebola Viral Disease 6
1.8 Influenza Virus Pandemic and Seasonal Influenza Outbreaks 8
1.9 Role of Environment in Influenza Virus Outbreaks 8
1.10 Middle East Respiratory Syndrome (MERS) 9
1.11 Severe Acute Respiratory Syndrome (SARS) 10
1.12 Environmental Factors That Influence SARS-CoV-2 Outbreaks 10
1.13 Detection and Prevention of Future Pandemics 12
 1.13.1 Continuous Surveillance 12
1.14 Conclusion 12
References 13

1.1 INTRODUCTION

Human existence and development cannot be considered without mentioning the impacts of pandemics and sporadic disease outbreaks in the environment, which typically comprises the physical, biological, social, and cultural factors that impact the lives of organisms in a particular setting, as humans are an integral part of the environment (Landon, 2006). Hence, any threat to lives is

DOI: 10.1201/9781003288732-1

a threat to the environment. Endemic diseases, outbreaks, epidemics, and pandemics have threatened humans, animals, and plants from time immemorial. From the time of plague, influenza, smallpox, meningitis, and cholera, to Human Immunodeficiency Virus (HIV)/acquired immunodeficiency syndrome (AIDS), severe acute respiratory syndrome coronavirus (SARS-CoV) and Middle East respiratory syndrome coronavirus (MERS-CoV), malaria, Ebola, Lassa fever, and in contemporary times COVID-19 and lately monkeypox, these diseases have had adverse consequences for humans and their environment. Indeed, these consequences have ranged from discontent to health deterioration to restrictions and a crash in the global economy (Piret and Boivin, 2021; WHO, 2022b).

In most cases, disease outbreaks have lasting impacts on the environment, including humans, as recovery takes a while. The environmental effects of infectious disease outbreaks can be overwhelming, depending on the response of the affected population. A disease occurrence can be categorised as endemic, an outbreak, epidemic, or pandemic based on its rate of transmission or spread in relation to the geographical areas reached (Grennan, 2019). Endemic diseases occur at an expected rate within a population, while an outbreak shows an unexpected rise in the number of people affected or in the occurrence of cases in a new environment. A disease outbreak is termed epidemic when it spreads widely, covering a broader area, while a pandemic is an epidemic with a global reach (Morens et al., 2004; Piret and Boivin, 2021). Viruses are primarily sustained in the environment through their interaction with their hosts and other environmental materials, such as binding to biofilms, sewage, and water bodies. However, these environments support the survival of non-enveloped viruses rather than enveloped ones with lipid coats, which are inactivated rapidly (Moresco et al., 2022). Pandemics have been part of human history dating back to the early 20th century (1918), when the Spanish flu claimed tens of millions of lives; it remains the most devastating pandemic (UNAIDS, 2018). Several other outbreaks have occurred since then with different magnitudes and impacts.

Disease outbreaks are heavy burdens on humanity, as many have no identified source, no established mode of transmission, and no symptoms, with a limiting effect on preventive measures. In any environment, the extent of an outbreak may be devastating due to its unprecedented nature. No environment exposed to a disease outbreak ever remains the same, irrespective of the cause. However, controlling such an outbreak may depend on how well the causative agent is understood. Studies have shown that most infectious diseases resulting in pandemics are caused by zoonotic pathogens that enter the human population through direct or indirect contact with animals, especially wildlife, through gaming, hunting, and international trade (Piret and Boivin, 2021). Understanding the mechanisms of pathogens' transmission to humans enables the establishment of novel methods to prevent and control infections.

Viruses are major culprits in disease outbreaks and those of a pandemic nature. The ability of a virus to cause a pandemic lies in its unique nature, being a sub-microscopic, obligate intracellular parasite containing genetic material surrounded by a protein coat (Chambers et al., 2020), and its ability to replicate in living cells and eventually cause a productive disease by its continuous production of new virions that can infect other cells in a host (Wolff et al., 2020). This sustained replication in the host and steady transmission enables the virus to acquire some genetic variation (mutation) that may enhance its transmissibility or infectiousness, leading to a pandemic (Drake and Holland, 1999). The host can be an animal or plant reservoir. Viruses that can jump from animals to humans, and enhanced ability to spread, even from human to human, can result in a pandemic (Parish et al., 2014). RNA viruses have been particularly implicated in previous and present pandemics, mainly due to their high mutation rate and ability to exist as variants, a unique feature of most pandemic viruses (Drake and Holland, 1999). Generally, pandemics have devastating impacts on individuals, communities, and societies across the world when they occur.

1.2 GLOBAL TREND OF VIRAL DISEASE OUTBREAKS

Viral diseases with pandemic potential mainly originate from animals known as non-human reservoirs, which may include arthropods, farm animals, and wild animals, including primates, rodents, and wild birds. Human infections occur due to interaction with these animals in their natural environment, climate change, and viral evolution that involves crossing between species, resulting in the emergence of novel viruses (Ippolito and Rezza, 2017). Notably, the pattern of disease outbreaks of viral origin across the globe started with H1N1 influenza or 'Spanish flu' of 1918, which claimed millions of lives (Patrono et al., 2022), and since then, numerous other disease outbreaks have occurred, including the current COVID-19. The history of pandemics has been reviewed extensively (Piret and Boivin, 2021; Baise et al., 2014; Harder and Werner, 2006; Jester et al., 2020)

1.3 HUMAN IMMUNODEFICIENCY VIRUS (HIV)/ACQUIRED IMMUNODEFICIENCY SYNDROME (AIDS)

AIDS is the end stage of HIV infection and a global pandemic first identified in 1981. It is due to infection by two genetically diverse isolates of the Lentivirus genus, namely HIV-1 and HIV-2 in the family Retroviridae, which initially infected non-human primates (simian immunodeficiency viruses) but spread to humans through cross-species transmission (Sharp and Hahn, 2011; Bbosa et al., 2019). HIV is said to have originated in the Democratic Republic of Congo and has spread globally (Faria et al., 2014; Bbosa et al., 2019). The two distinct genotypes of the virus HIV-1 gave rise to several other groups or serotypes, M (Major), O (Outlier), N (non-M, non-O), and P, which show a degree of specific geographical distribution. HIV-2 has about nine subtypes or groups (A to I) (Sharp and Hahn, 2011; Visseaux et al., 2016).

HIV-1 is widespread and has been reported globally. Subtype B is prevalent mainly in Europe and the Americas, while M subtypes have global dominance. The remaining groups, N, O, and P, are distributed geographically. HIV-2 remains predominant in West Africa but has also been reported in some parts of Europe, including France and Portugal. Other countries where HIV-2 has been reported include India and the US (Visseaux et al., 2016). HIV, irrespective of type, circulates widely and according to United Nations Programme on HIV/AIDS (UNAIDS) (2018), has had an unimaginably catastrophic impact on humans in modern history, leading to 77.3 million infections and 35.4 million deaths worldwide as of December 2017 (UNAIDS, 2018).

The scourge of the HIV/AIDS pandemic started in 1981 (UNAIDS, 2018) and particularly hit the developing nations, including sub-Saharan Africa, where the poor standard of living and lack of access to adequate healthcare services aggravated the outcome of the disease in infected populations (WHO, 2020).

1.4 HIV/AIDS EPIDEMIOLOGY AND IMPACTS IN AFRICA

Africa alone recorded an estimated 1.8 million new HIV infections in 2009 (UNAIDS, 2010), accounting for about 68–69% of new infections worldwide. In addition, in previous years, about 390,000 infected children, mainly through mother-to-child transmission, had been recorded (UNAIDS, 2010; UNAIDS and WHO, 2009); however, a year or two later, the number decreased to about 370,000 new infections after the initiation of antiretroviral therapy in the region (UNAIDS, 2010).

Over 1.3 million Africans had lost their lives to AIDS as of 2009 (UNAIDS, 2010). Also, the number of orphaned children increased, as an estimated 14.8 million had lost one or both parents to AIDS at that time (UNAIDS, 2010).

In 2018, about 25.7 million people were living with HIV in Africa; there were 1.1 million new infections and 470,000 deaths from AIDS-related illnesses. In West and Central Africa, sexual partners accounted for 64% of new HIV infections and 25% of new HIV infections in the East and Southern African subregion (WHO, 2018b).

The devastating impact of the HIV/AIDS pandemic ranges from severe losses, including economic and developmental, to a direct negative effect on the total gross domestic product (GDP). The pandemic severely affected four important critical sectors in the continent: African development, health, the state, and academia. This was a result of the high burden of infection in the region (Institute of Medicine Committee, 2011). There was severe loss of life among young adults, who made up the workforce and had millions of dependents; this subsequently led to food insecurity due to poor agricultural engagement, loss of social safety nets, and resultant abject poverty, with an increased number of vulnerable populations in the region (Commission on HIV/AIDS and Governance in Africa, 2008). However, due to the introduction of antiretroviral therapy through the efforts of national HIV programmes and other international partners and civil society groups, HIV infections decreased by 37% between 2000 and 2018, resulting in a low rate of HIV-related deaths (WHO, 2018b).

In the recent past, while a tremendous effort has been made in the fight against HIV globally through the discovery and use of antiretroviral therapy and combination therapy for the treatment of HIV/AIDS patients (Staitieh et al., 2017), cure and elimination of the virus remain elusive, as the virus rebounds soon after interrupting therapy (Nixon et al., 2017). As a result, there is a severe decline in HIV service delivery, which varies by country or region but is seen more in developing countries due to the termination of most national and international HIV programmes. In 2019, global deaths from HIV were estimated at 690,000, while new HIV infections were estimated at 1.7 million (WHO, 2020). These new infections account for more than 62% of the HIV burden, especially among young people globally, between the ages of 15 and 49 years, in 2019 alone (Benton et al., 2019; WHO, 2020). A large population of people living with HIV (PLWH) resides in low- and middle-income countries, especially in sub-Saharan Africa, with more than 68% of the global infection. This challenge now becomes compounded by the sudden emergence of SARS-CoV-2, responsible for the present pandemic, which has not only impacted global health but also adversely affected the socio-economic growth of nations (Fernandes, 2020). Furthermore, the impact of COVID-19 on the HIV pandemic has affected HIV research, diagnosis, and treatment of patients, and this trend may persist even after the COVID-19 pandemic is over, because the aftermath of these concurrent pandemics (SARS-CoV-2 and HIV) will continue to linger (Chenneville et al., 2020).

1.5 RELATIONSHIP BETWEEN HIV/AIDS AND THE ENVIRONMENT

A couple of factors are considered when linking the HIV/AIDS pandemic and the environment. These include effects of climate change, migration of the human population, and availability of food and water (Bloem et al., 2010) and other natural resources (Talman et al., 2013). The environment plays a significant role in the epidemiology of HIV/AIDS and the disease outcome in vulnerable populations. Sub-Saharan Africa is one of the regions most badly hit by the HIV pandemic, where a series of environmental changes emanating from climate change has been observed in rural communities. In addition, most of these places have depleting natural resources, resulting in massive human migration due to conflicts, poverty, and inequality, hence driving and sustaining the spread and outcomes of disease in these regions (Hunter et al., 2011; Talman et al., 2013). Typically, environmental degradation and pollution have adverse effects on the course of diseases, including HIV/AIDS. A filthy environment and increased influx of toxic substances into the ecosystem compromise healthy individuals' immune systems and may reduce infected persons' coping strength (Bolton and Talman, 2010).

Dependence on natural resources may also be an outcome of HIV/AIDS, which may emanate from the loss of the workforce due to the pandemic, as observed in most communities ravaged by the disease where many children were left as orphans (Benton et al., 2019). In addition, the livelihood of these vulnerable populations may be adversely affected, as risky behaviours such as promiscuity and substance abuse that increase the spread of HIV may predispose them to HIV vulnerability (Bolton and Talman, 2010).

However, further studies are needed to adequately quantify the effects of the HIV/AIDS pandemic on the environment and vice versa in the regions most affected, including the African region.

1.6 EBOLA VIRAL DISEASE OUTBREAK AND RE-EMERGENCE

Recently, viral haemorrhagic diseases have increased in Africa, caused by viruses in the *Arenaviridae*, *Bunyaviridae*, *Flaviviridae*, and *Filoviridae* families. In most cases, the environment plays a major role, as animal reservoirs have been implicated in the emergence of these viruses and sustained transmission to the human population (Shenge and Opayele, 2020). Ebola virus is one such virus, which causes severe haemorrhagic fever in humans. The African continent and the entire globe are at the risk of experiencing Ebola disease as a pandemic. The virus has existed on the continent for decades. The virus causes haemorrhagic fever and belongs to the *Filoviridae* family and the order Mononegavirales (Baise et al., 2014). Several reports have noted the circulation of this virus among monkeys and chimpanzees in the forest zones of the Democratic Republic of Congo (DRC) (WHO, 2018d). However, human infection was not recorded until 1976, when the initial outbreaks co-occurred in the remote areas of these countries (WHO, 2021). The index case of the Ebola viral disease outbreak occurred in remote villages in Central Africa, near tropical rainforests. Between 2014 and 2016, an outbreak occurred in West Africa, the largest and most complex Ebola outbreak since the virus was first discovered in 1976 (WHO, 2021). Several Ebola disease outbreaks were reported, with more than 28,000 cases and over 11,000 deaths recorded in Liberia, Guinea, Sierra Leone, the DRC, and Nigeria (Baise et al., 2014; Shenge and Opayele, 2020). Ebola is an ecological disease, typically transmitted to humans from wild animals, including fruit bats, porcupines, and primates, especially to hunters and handlers, who then spread it to other individuals, primarily through direct contact with the blood and body secretions, organs, or other bodily fluids of infected persons. Infection can also occur through contaminated surfaces or materials, including clothing, bedding, and objects that have been in contact with contaminated body fluids (WHO, 2021).

1.7 ENVIRONMENTAL IMPACT OF EBOLA VIRAL DISEASE

Ebola outbreaks in the African environment have caused numerous deaths (fatalities) ranging from 25% to 90% during the past outbreaks and have spread to other countries such as Guinea and across land borders to Sierra Leone and Liberia (WHO, 2021). According to the World Health Organization (WHO) (2021), the sequence of outbreaks in the region started with the case in West Africa between 2014 and 2016; Bas-Uele, DRC (May–July, 2017); Equateur, DRC (May–July, 2018); North Kivu/Ituri, DRC (August 2018–June 2020); N'Zerekore, Guinea (February–June 2021); North Kivu, DRC (February–May, 2021); North Kivu, DRC (October–December, 2021); and it has re-emerged in the year 2022 (WHO, 2021).

Re-emergence, however, has posed some pertinent questions that may lead to understanding the biology of Ebola and its sustenance in the environment. What could be responsible for the sudden re-emergence of this virus 38 years after decades of hibernation? Could socio-ecological and epidemiological factors be accountable for adaptation and transmission of Ebola virus in the region? How does the global insight and response to this present epidemic affect the spread and possible future outbreaks? Until the 2014 outbreak, little was known about Ebola disease in the general African population, though it has existed for years. Over several years, the gap in knowledge and surveillance of the disease promoted primary transmission among rural, semi-urban, and urban dwellers, influencing the establishment of the disease and cross-border transmission among West African countries and beyond (WHO, 2021). In addition, the disease has the potential to become a global pandemic based on the current trend of steady re-emergence. According to Redding et al. (2019), modelling results suggest future Ebola disease outbreaks in West and Central Africa, following an analysis of disease drivers of Ebola disease risks. Their modelling study reported an increase of 1.75–3.2 in the disease rate at the interface of animal–human–virus circulation in Africa by 2070 (Redding et al., 2019).

Environmental factors such as climate change can affect a pathogen's life cycle and its adaptation in any environment, including time and rate of transmission, mode of spread of the virus, and the species involved (Daouda et al., 2015). In addition, population migration, as well as vector habitation, can influence Ebola disease outcomes. Environmental drivers of Ebola disease outbreak or emergence typically are connected to ecosystem modifications due to climate change, human–animal interactions resulting in zoonoses, an ecological adaptation of animal reservoirs, including bats, monkeys, and other wild animal species involved in Ebola virus transmission, and socio-economic factors (Daouda et al., 2015; Redding et al., 2019).

Typically, adequate knowledge about the ecology of the Ebola virus, human population behaviour, and the impact of climate change on viral transmission and epidemiology will play a significant role in Ebola prevention, control, and eradication. However, misinformation of the general public through inadequate research into some social, economic, and scientific factors supporting Ebola re-emergence will pose a more serious global challenge. Ebola virus is a class 4 pathogen (deadly); hence, strict safety measures must follow in any environment wherever and whenever Ebola is suspected. Safety is the key to prevention and control.

Creating awareness through educational public health messages about the risk factors for the disease and measures people can take to protect themselves is vital in reducing infection and deaths associated with Ebola. Therefore, there is a need for integrated, continuous participatory surveillance to better understand the epidemiology and pathogenesis of Ebola and to mount preventive and control strategies against this deadly disease of public health significance with pandemic potential.

1.8 INFLUENZA VIRUS PANDEMIC AND SEASONAL INFLUENZA OUTBREAKS

According to WHO, a six-stage classification has outlined the course of infection by a novel influenza virus that can lead to a pandemic. The initial stage may involve an influenza virus strain that mostly infects animals or emanates from animal reservoirs; the animals infect humans later on, or vice versa; then, through direct infection between humans, it can lead to a pandemic (WHO, 2009a).

Influenza virus disease ('flu') was first recognised nearly simultaneously across continents in the summer of 1918; then, it peaked in the autumn of 1918 (Morens et al., 2007) and continued through the winter of 1919 (Patrono et al., 2022). During the pandemic, young children and the elderly were severely affected, and the 1918 pandemic caused exceptionally high mortality in healthy populations aged between 20 and 40 years (The Malaysian Insider, 2009). In addition, the duration of the pandemic, characterised by high mortality and an unusual disease course, contributed to its unprecedented impact on the human population at that time. Consequently, all the other influenza virus outbreaks, such as H1N2, H2N2, and H3N2, are descendants of the H1N1 Spanish flu of 1918 (Patrono et al., 2022). Figure 1.1 shows the major strains of influenza viruses in circulation, differentiated by the number of haemagglutinin and neuraminidase viral proteins.

1.9 ROLE OF ENVIRONMENT IN INFLUENZA VIRUS OUTBREAKS

Typically, the persistence of influenza virus in the environment depends on climatic variations in atmospheric temperature, humidity, salinity, pH, air pollution levels, and to some extent, solar radiations (Sooryanarain and Elankumaran, 2015). Among these environmental factors, temperature and humidity largely influence the spread of influenza virus, especially cool-dry weather conditions, which facilitate virus attachment in the respiratory tract and virus transmissibility (Sooryanarain and Elankumaran, 2015). In particular, tropical and subtropical zones exhibit slight seasonal differences. For example, high-altitude regions experience outbreaks in temperate or cold climates, while outbreaks in low-latitude zones occur mostly during humid-rainy conditions. Influenza A and B viruses mainly cause seasonal epidemics in humans, especially during the cold seasons in temperate regions (Sooryanarain and Elankumaran, 2015).

Different strains of the influenza virus have emerged over time as a result of re-assortment of genes (shift and drift) and variations that occur in animal reservoirs, especially birds and swine, with major variants such as H1N1 (swine flu), H1N2, and H3N2, H5N1 (bird flu) now being detected in both humans and animal populations (Shenge and Opayele, 2020). As of 2009, about six major influenza epidemics had occurred in the last 140 years, with the Spanish flu of 1918 pandemic being the most severe due to the loss of about 50–100 million lives (WHO, 2009b).

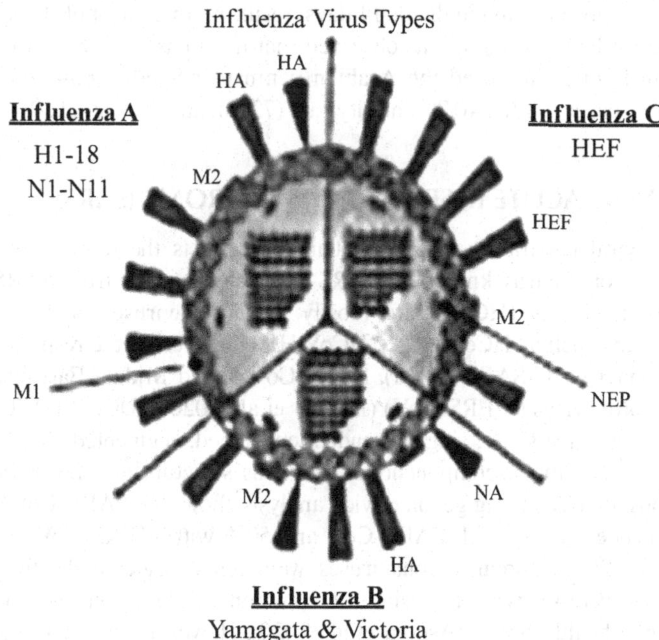

FIGURE 1.1 Schematic structure of influenza virus strains. (From Francis, M.E., et al., *Viruses*, 11, 122, 2019.)

In Africa, particularly in sub-Saharan Africa, circulation of classical avian, swine, or pandemic influenza has been established, although more understanding of the epidemiology of influenza virus in humans is needed in the region, as disease surveillance is poor (Elelu, 2017). For instance, in 2006, an outbreak of H5N1 (bird flu) led to the destruction of several million birds, with one recorded fatal human infection (Ekong et al., 2012). This was followed by an outbreak of highly pathogenic H1N1 (swine flu) in 2009 (Shenge and Opayele, 2020). Hence, more studies are needed to quantify the disease's economic and public health impacts in sub-Saharan Africa.

1.10 MIDDLE EAST RESPIRATORY SYNDROME (MERS)

The Middle East respiratory syndrome coronavirus (MERS-CoV) is a coronavirus responsible for the MERS epidemic, which was first isolated from a patient presenting with severe pneumonia in 2012 (Oh et al., 2018). The MERS-CoV outbreaks seemed to have affected mainly the Middle East region and some Asian countries (WHO, 2018c). The disease was said to have spread from individuals who, at the time, had visited many medical settings, resulting in a series of infections presented as respiratory sequelae (Nishiura et al., 2016).

The outbreak in Korea in 2015 involved 186 cases, causing 38 fatalities (Oh et al., 2018; Nishiura et al., 2016). However, the MERS-CoV outbreak was contained by isolating exposed individuals for 14 days, resulting in control of the spread of the disease (WHO, 2018c). It was observed that most cases of MERS-CoV that occurred in humans involved the Arabian peninsula; Saudi Arabia recorded a total of 1,783 cases, with a 40.7% fatality rate (726 deaths) (Oh et al., 2018).

1.11 SEVERE ACUTE RESPIRATORY SYNDROME (SARS)

SARS is a viral respiratory disease that mainly affects the respiratory system, caused by a coronavirus known as SARS-associated coronavirus (SARS-CoV). Human coronaviruses (HCoVs) are mostly betacoronaviruses, and this group includes strains such as HCoV-OC43, HCoV-HKU1, severe acute respiratory syndrome coronavirus 1 (SARS-CoV-1), SARS-CoV-2, and Middle East respiratory syndrome coronavirus (MERS-CoV) (Dilcher et al., 2020; CDC, 2017). The virus consists of a positive-sense, single-stranded, enveloped, segmented RNA genome (CDC, 2017). The major components of the virus structure are shown in Figure 1.2. Previous analyses using genome-wide analysis show that SARS-CoV-2 shares 79.5% sequence identity with SARS-CoV and 50% with MERS-CoV (Jin et al., 2020). As of 2002, human coronaviruses were not considered deadly viruses, because they were known for causing the common cold and were not viewed as serious public health threats (Ashour et al., 2020). However, this view changed in early 2003 when the disease occurred in Asia in February 2003, and in the same period spread to over 29 countries in 4 continents, including North America, South America, Europe, and Asia. The SARS-CoV-1 outbreak resulted in 8,422 infections and 916 deaths (WHO, 2020; CDC, 2017). In 2019, a novel coronavirus strain named 2019-new coronavirus (2019-nCoV) emerged in Wuhan, China, and was declared a pandemic on 11 March 2020. However, the virus was later renamed 'severe acute respiratory syndrome coronavirus 2' (SARS-CoV-2) after discovering that the virus was in the same family as the previous strain (SARS-CoV-1) (WHO, 2020).

The SARS-CoV-2 outbreak has numerous impacts on the environment. As of 20 May 2022, 6,274,323 deaths had occurred due to SARS-CoV-2 disease (WHO, 2022b). The impact of COVID-19 was felt most during the global lockdown to control the spread of the virus. The socio-economic, environmental, and psychological well-being of individuals have been seriously affected by SARS-CoV-2 pandemics, especially in developing countries, where the quality of life is at the barest minimum (WHO, 2022a). Furthermore, the SARS-CoV-2 virus persists in the environment, which may affect its elimination. Studies have reported the persistence of the virus in different environments. For instance, the virus persists and is transmitted through aerosols (Ge et al., 2020), fomites, and environmental surfaces (China News, 2020).

1.12 ENVIRONMENTAL FACTORS THAT INFLUENCE SARS-COV-2 OUTBREAKS

The transmission and survival of most enveloped and non-enveloped viruses may depend on certain environmental features. SARS-CoV-2 persists in

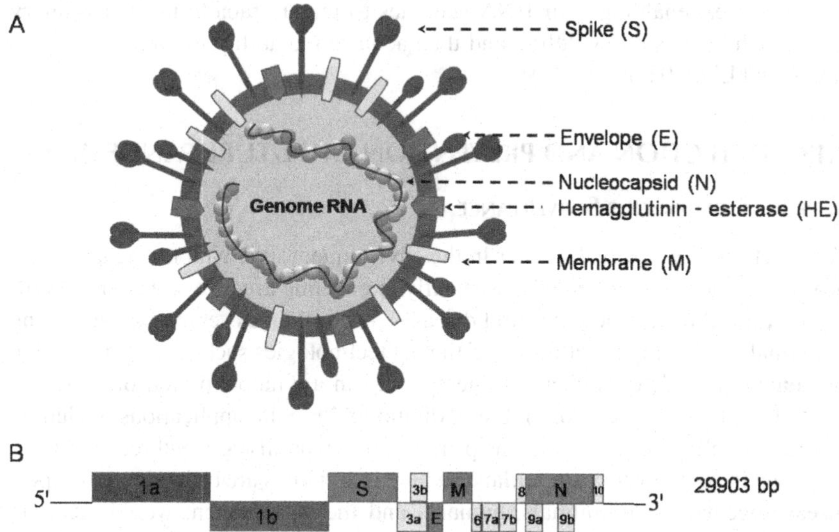

FIGURE 1.2 Electron micrograph of Coronavirus particle, indicating the major viral components. (From Jin, Y, et al., *Viruses*, 27, 372, 2020.)

aerosols and is transmitted as droplets suspended in the air. Hence, poor air quality, including in enclosed buildings, may facilitate the spread of the virus (Azuma et al., 2020). Furthermore, other important materials that can sustain the virus at room temperature for about 2 to 4 days include door knobs, stainless steel, plastics, and glass surfaces (Azuma et al., 2020). The ability of the virus to survive on fomites for days and its transmission through droplets is one reason why the outbreak spread quickly and became a pandemic in a very short period. SARS-CoV-2 has been reported in wastewater and effluents from sewage tanks contaminated by the virus. Medical wastes dumped at land sites and into the ocean and other water bodies are sources of infection in such environments, as humans and aquatic animals come in contact with these sources in one way or another (Saadat et al., 2020).

On the other hand, few studies have reported the presence of influenza virus and coronaviruses in sewage. The only limitation is the unstable nature of their lipid envelope, which can easily dissolve and be inactivated in the environment (Moresco et al., 2022). Again, harsh weather conditions such as extreme heat may equally affect the lipid envelope and render the virus inactive, as high temperature was demonstrated by Biryukov et al. (2021) to increase the rate of degeneration of SARS-CoV-2 on surfaces and other fomites (Biryukov et al., 2021).

MERS-CoV and SARS-CoV are similar in many ways. These include the ability of both viruses to infect animals and humans, causing zoonotic infection, which is characteristic of coronaviruses as they constantly evolve (Zhou et al., 2021). This results from recombination processes, which appear to be frequent in coronaviruses, enabling their RNA genomes to mutate rapidly in their primary hosts, such as bats and wildlife, and then acquire the ability to jump to humans (Fung and Liu, 2021).

1.13 DETECTION AND PREVENTION OF FUTURE PANDEMICS

1.13.1 Continuous Surveillance

To detect disease outbreaks faster in the environment, it is vital to engage public health agencies and individuals, especially in endemic areas, in constant surveillance of novel or re-emerging viral diseases. A continuous screening and testing of animals and humans with state-of-the-art technologies such as next-generation sequencing that detect infectious agents, even in a window period of infection, is needed (Shenge et al., 2020). Using digital and mobile applications, including artificial intelligence, may also help track infectious disease outbreaks. Again, engaging in participatory surveillance where individuals are trained to self-report disease occurrence in animals, humans, and the environment would facilitate early detection of infectious disease epidemics. In remote communities, especially in sub-Saharan Africa, where some rural settings are hard to reach, implementing integrated programmes such as awareness of infectious disease epidemics, transmission cycle, and prevention at the grass roots may be helpful. Detection of diseases with pandemic potential requires a collective effort whereby all stakeholders, including governmental, private, and civil society groups, get involved in processes that will succeed in detecting and curtailing epidemic threats in an environment. The inclusion of global surveillance programmes and best practices in determining diseases of pandemic potential among animals and zoonotic pathogens, water-borne pathogens, and vector-borne diseases may be of paramount importance to rapidly detect the emergence of infectious threats through the sources described earlier.

1.14 CONCLUSION

This chapter has discussed the basic features of the various viral disease outbreaks, of which some have had global spread. The environment plays a major role in infectious disease outbreaks; hence, understanding the One Health approach (human–animal–environment) to disease occurrence, transmission, and re-emergence is paramount. As pandemics affect every facet of human development, there is a need for increased effort in prevention. This requires global collaborations between and among nations, encompassing governments, public–private partnerships, and philanthropic efforts to support projects and ideas that will culminate in prevention of or rapid response to outbreaks. Given this, novel technologies should be made available for rapid diagnostic testing, contact tracing, disease biomarker identification, and new platforms for designing and producing effective vaccines to prepare for an effective response in future pandemics.

REFERENCES

Ashour HM, Elkhatib WF, Rahman M, Elshabrawy HA (2020). Insights into the recent 2019 novel coronavirus (SARS-CoV-2) in light of past human coronavirus outbreaks. *Pathogens*; 9(3): 18.

Azuma K, Yanagi U, Kagi N, Kim H, Ogata M, Hayashi M (2020). Environmental factors involved in SARS-CoV-2 transmission: Effect and role of indoor environmental quality in the strategy for COVID-19 infection control. *Environ Health Prev Med*; 25(1): 66. doi: 10.1186/s12199-020-00904-2.

Baize S, Pannetier D, Oestereich L, Rieger T, Koivogui L, Magassouba N, Soropogui B, Sow MS, Keïta S, De Clerck H, Tiffany A, Dominguez G, Loua M, Traoré A, Kolié M, Malano ER, Heleze E, Bocquin A, Mély S, Raoul H, Caro V, Cadar D, Gabriel M, Pahlmann M, Tappe D, Schmidt-Chanasit J, Impouma B, Diallo AK, Formenty P, Van Herp M, Günther S (2014). Emergence of Zaire Ebola virus disease in guinea. *N Engl J Med*; 371(15): 1418–1425. doi: 10.1056/NEJMoa1404505.

Bbosa N, Kaleebu PB, Ssemwanga D (2019). HIV subtype diversity worldwide. *Curr Opin HIV AIDS*; 14(3): 153–160. doi: 10.1097/COH.0000000000000534.

Benton TD, Kee Ng WY, Leung D, Canetti A, Karnik N (2019). Depression among youth living with HIV/AIDS. *Child Adolesc Psychiatr Clin N Am*; 28(3): 447–459. doi: 10.1016/j.chc.2019.02.014.

Biryukov J, Boydston JA, Dunning RA, Yeager JJ, Wood S, Ferris A, Miller D, Weaver W, Zeitouni NE, Freeburger D, Dabisch P, Wahl V, Hevey MC, Altamura LA (2021). SARS-CoV-2 is rapidly inactivated at high temperature. *Environ Chem Lett*; 19(2): 1773–1777. doi: 10.1007/s10311-021-01187-x.

Bloem MW, Semba RD, Kraemer K (2010). Castel Gandolfo workshop: An introduction to the impact of climate change, the economic crisis, and the increase in the food prices on malnutrition. *J Nutr*; 140(1): 132S–135S. doi: 10.3945/jn.109.112094.

Bolton S, Talman A (2010). *Interactions between HIV/AIDS and the Environment: A Review of the Evidence and Recommendations for Next Steps*. Nairobi, Kenya: IUCN ESARO.

Chambers JP, Yu J, Valdes JJ, Arulanandam BP (2020). SARS-CoV-2, early entry events. *J Pathog*; 2020: 11. doi: 10.1155/2020/9238696.

Centers for disease Control and Prevention, CDC (2017). Severe acute respiratory syndrome (SARS). Available online at: https://www.cdc.gov/sars/index.html. Accessed May 15, 2022.

Chenneville T, Gabbidon K, Hanson P, Holyfield C (2020). The impact of COVID-19 on HIV treatment and research: A call to action. *Int J Environ Res Public Health*; 17(12): 4548. doi: 10.3390/ijerph17124548.

China News (2020). [The SARS-COV-2 nucleic acid detected for the first time on the surface of door handle in Guangzhou and cleaning taken attention]. https://www.msn.com/zh-tw/news/world. Accessed May 16, 2020.

Commission on HIV/AIDS and Governance in Africa (2008). Securing our future: Report of the commission on HIV/AIDS and Governance in Africa. Archived Resource. uneca.org.

Daouda K, Mathieu B, François R (2015). Climate change and Ebola outbreaks: Are they connected? In *Our Common Future under Climate Change*. International Scientific Conference Abstract Book 7–10 July 2015. Paris, France.

Dilcher M, Werno A, Jennings LC (2020). SARS-CoV-2: A novel deadly virus in a globalised world. *N Z Med J*; 133(1510): 6.

Drake JW, Holland JJ (1999). Mutation rates among RNA viruses. *PNAS*; 96(24): 13910–13913. doi: 10.1073/pnas.96.24.13910.

Elelu N (2017). Epidemiological risk factors of knowledge and preventive practice regarding avian influenza among poultry farmers and live bird traders in Ikorodu, Lagos State, Nigeria. *Int J Vet Sci Med*; 5(1): 47–52. doi: 10.1016/j.ijvsm.2017.03.002.

Ekong PS, Ducheyne E, Carpenter TE, Owolodu AT, Lombin LH, Berkvens D (2012). Spatio-temporal epidemiology of highly pathogenic avian influenza (H5N1) outbreaks in Nigeria, 2006–2008. *Prev Vet Med*; 103(2–3): 170–177.

Faria NR, Rambaut A, Suchard MA, Baele G, Bedford T, Ward MJ, Tatem AJ, Sousa JD, Arinaminpathy N, Pépin J, Posada D, Peeters M, Pybus OG, Lemey P (2014). The early spread and epidemic ignition of HIV-1 in human populations. *Science*; 346(6205): 56–61.

Fernandes N (2020). Economic effects of coronavirus outbreak (COVID-19) on the world economy. *SSRN Journal*; 2020. doi: 10.2139/ssrn.3557504.

Fung TS, Liu DX (2021). Similarities and dissimilarities of COVID-19 and other coronavirus diseases. *Annu Rev Microbiol*; 75: 19–47. doi: 10.1146/annurev-micro-110520-023212.

Francis ME, King ML, Kelvin AA (2019). Back to the future for influenza preimmunity – Looking back at influenza virus history to infer the outcome of future infections. *Viruses*; 11(2): 122. doi: 10.3390/v11020122.

Ge ZY, Yang LM, Xia J-J, Fu XH, Zhang YZ (2020). Possible aerosol transmission of COVID-19 and special precautions in dentistry. *J Zhejiang Univ Sci B*; 21(5): 361–368.

Grennan D (2019). What is a pandemic? *JAMA*; 321(9): 910. doi: 10.1001/jama.2019.0700.

Harder TC, Werner O (2006). Avian influenza. In Kamps BS, Hoffman C, Preiser W (eds.), *Influenza Report 2006*. Paris: Flying Publisher, 48–88.

Hunter LM, Twine W, Johnson A (2011). Adult mortality and natural resource use in rural South Africa: Evidence from the Agincourt health and demographic surveillance site. *Soc Nat Resour*; 24(3): 256–275. doi: 10.1080/08941920903443327.

Institute of Medicine (US) Committee on Envisioning a Strategy for the Long-Term Burden of HIV/AIDS: African Needs and US Interests (2011). *Preparing for the Future of HIV/AIDS in Africa: A Shared Responsibility*. Washington, DC: National Academies Press (US). 4, The Burden of HIV/AIDS: Implications for African States and Societies. Available from https://www.ncbi.nlm.nih.gov/books/NBK209743/.

Ippolito G, Rezza G (2017). Preface - Emerging viruses: From early detection to intervention. *Adv Exp Med Biol*; 972: 1–5. doi: 10.1007/5584_2017_33.

Jester BJ, Uyeki TM, Jernigan DB (2020). Fifty years of influenza A(H3N2) following the pandemic of 1968. *Am J Public Health*; 110(5): 669–676. doi: 10.2105/AJPH.2019.305557.

Jin Y, Yang H, Ji W, Wu W, Chen S, Zhang W, Duan G (2020). Virology, epidemiology, pathogenesis, and control of COVID-19. *Viruses*; 27(4): 372. doi: 10.3390/v12040372.

Landon M (2006). *Environment, Health and Sustainable Development*. Open University Press, 1–213.

Morens DM, Folkers GK, Fauci AS (2004). The challenge of emerging and re-emerging infectious diseases. *Nature*; 430(6996): 242–249. doi: 10. 1038/nature02759.

Morens DM, Fauci AS (2007). The 1918 influenza pandemic: Insights for the 21st century. *J Infect Dis*; 195(7): 1018–1028. doi: 10.1086/511989.

Moresco V, Charatzidou A, Oliver DM, Weidmann M, Matallana-Surget S, Quilliam RS (2022). Binding, recovery, and infectiousness of enveloped and non-enveloped viruses associated with plastic pollution in surface water. *Environ Pollut*; 308: 119594. doi: 10.1016/j.envpol.2022.119594.

Nishiura H, Endo A, Saitoh M, Kinoshita R, Ueno R, Nakaoka S, Miyamatsu Y, Dong Y, Chowell G, Mizumoto K (2016). Identifying determinants of heterogeneous transmission dynamics of the Middle East respiratory syndrome (MERS) outbreak in the Republic of Korea, 2015: A retrospective epidemiological analysis. *BMJ (Open)*; 6(2): e009936. doi: 10.1136/bmjopen-2015-009936.

Nixon CC, Mavigner M, Silvestri G, Garcia JV (2017). In vivo models of human immunodeficiency virus persistence and cure strategies. *J Infect Dis*; 215(suppl_3): S142–S151. doi: 10.1093/infdis/jiw637.

Oh MD, Park WB, Park SW, Choe PG, Bang JH, Song KH, Kim ES, Kim HB, Kim NJ (2018). Middle East respiratory syndrome: What we learned from the 2015 outbreak in the Republic of Korea. *Korean J Intern Med*; 33(2): 233–246. doi: 10.3904/kjim.2018.031.

Parish IA, Marshall HD, Staron MM, Lang PA, Brüstle A, Chen JH, Cui W, Tsui YC, Perry C, Laidlaw BJ, Ohashi PS, Weaver CT, Kaech SM (2014). Chronic viral infection promotes sustained Th1-derived immunoregulatory IL-10 via BLIMP-1. *J Clin Invest*; 124(8): 3455–3468. doi: 10.1172/JCI66108.

Patrono LV, Vrancken B, Budt M, Düx A, Lequime S, Boral S, Gilbert MTP, Gogarten JF, Hoffmann L, Horst D, Merkel K, Morens D, Prepoint B, Schlotterbeck J, Schuenemann VJ, Suchard MA, Taubenberger JK, Tenkhoff L, Urban C, Widulin N, Winter E, Worobey M, Schnalke T, Wolff T, Lemey P, Calvignac-Spencer S (2022). Archival influenza virus genomes from Europe reveal genomic variability during the 1918 pandemic. *Nat Commun*; 13(1): 2314. doi: 10.1038/s41467-022-29614-9.

Piret J, Boivin G (2021). Pandemics throughout history. *Front Microbiol*; 11: 631736. doi: 10.3389/fmicb.2020.631736.

Redding DW, Atkinson PM, Cunningham AA, Iacono GL, Moses LM, Wood JLN, Jones KE (2019). Impacts of environmental and socio-economic factors on emergence and epidemic potential of Ebola in Africa. *Nat Commun*; 10(1): 4531. doi: 10.1038/s41467-019-12499-6.

Saadat S, Rawtani D, Hussain CM (2020). Environmental perspective of COVID-19. *Sci Total Environ*; 728: 138870. doi: 10.1016/j.scitotenv.2020.138870.

Sharp PM, Hahn BH (2011). Origins of HIV and the AIDS pandemic. *Cold Spring Harb Perspect Med*; 1(1): a006841.

Shenge JA, Opayele AV (2020). The impact and control of emerging and re-emerging viral diseases in the environment: An African perspective. In *Current Microbiological Research in Africa*, pp. 185–202. doi: 10.1007/978-3-030-35296-7_7.

Staitieh BS, Egea EE, Guidot DM (2017). Pulmonary innate immune dysfunction in human immunodeficiency virus. *Am J Respir Cell Mol Biol*; 56(5): 563–567. doi: 10.1165/rcmb.2016-0213TR.

Sooryanarain H, Elankumaran S (2015). Environmental role in influenza virus outbreaks. *Annu Rev Anim Biosci*; 3: 347–373. doi: 10.1146/annurev-animal-022114-111017.

Talman A, Bolton S, Walson JL (2013). Interactions between HIV/AIDS and the environment: Toward a syndemic framework. *Am J Public Health*; 103(2): 253–261. doi: 10.2105/AJPH.2012.300924.

The Malaysian Insider (2009). *H1N1 Fatality Rates Comparable to Seasonal Flu.* Washington, DC. Reuters. Archived from the original on October 20, 2009. Retrieved May 5, 2022.

UNAIDS (2018). Facts sheet-world AIDS day 2018. *2030 Ending the AIDS https://www.unaids.org/en/resources/documents/2018/JC2686_WAD2018report. Epidemic.*

UNAIDS and WHO (2009). *AIDS Epidemic Update: December 2009.* Geneva: UNAIDS.

UNAIDS (The Joint United Nations Programme on HIV/AIDS) (2010). *Global Report: UNAIDS Report on the Global AIDS Epidemic 2010.* Geneva: UNAIDS.

Visseaux B, Damond F, Matheron S, Descamps D, Charpentier C (2016). Hiv-2 molecular epidemiology. *Infect Genet Evol*; 46: 233–240.

Wolff G, Melia CE, Snijder EJ, Bárcena M (2020). Double-membrane vesicles as platforms for viral replication. *Trends Microbiol*; 28(12): 1022–1033. doi: 10.1016/j.tim.2020.05.009.

World Health Organization (2009a). *Pandemic Influenza Preparedness and Response: A WHO Guidance Document.* Geneva: World Health Organization; 2009. 4, THE WHO PANDEMIC PHASES. Available from: https://www.ncbi.nlm.nih.gov/books/NBK143061/ *Alert.*

World Health Organization (2009b). *World Now at the Start of 2009 Influenza.* , Dr Margaret Chan, Director-General of the World Health Organization, Geneva, 2009.11 June 2009 *Pandemic*

WHO (2009). Pandemic (H1N1) 2009 – Update 74. *Situation Updates – Pandemic (H1N1) 2009.* Archived from the original on November 15, 2009.

WHO (2018a). *Influenza: Fact Sheet 6.* Archived from the Original on December 17, 2019. Accessed May 4, 2022.

WHO (2018b). https://www.afro.who.int/health-topics/hivaids. Accessed May 10, 2022.

WHO (2018c). *Middle East Respiratory Syndrome Coronavirus (MERS-CoV)* [Internet] [cited 2018 February 8]. Geneva: World Health Organization. Available from http://who.int/emergencies/mers-cov/en/.

WHO (2018d). *Update on Ebola Outbreak and Emergency Preparedness and Response in DRC.* Accessed April 5, 2022.

WHO (2020). *Severe Acute Respiratory Syndrome.* http://www.emro.who.int/healthtopics/severe-acute-respiratory-syndrome/ Accessed May 15, 2022.

WHO (2021). Fact sheet. https://www.who.int/health-topics/ebola/. Accessed April 12, 2022.

WHO (2022a). https://www.cnbc.com/2022/05/20/world-health-organization-confirms-80-cases-of-monkeypox-with-outbreaks-in-11-countries.html.

WHO (2022b). Facts sheet. https//www.who.int/covid-19. Accessed May 13, 2022.

Zhou H, Yang J, Zhou C, Chen B, Fang H, Chen S, Zhang X, Wang L, Zhang L (2021). A review of SARS-CoV2: Compared with SARS-CoV and MERS-CoV. *Front Med (Lausanne)*; 7(8): 628370. doi: 10.3389/fmed.2021.628370.

2 Climate Change

Emerging Driver of Infectious Diseases

Ayukafangha Etando and Akebe Luther King Abia

CONTENTS

2.1 Introduction 17
2.2 Climate Change Factors Enhancing Infectious Disease Rate 18
 2.2.1 Anthropogenic Factors of Climate Change and Infectious Diseases 18
 2.2.2 Demographic Factors of Climate Change and Infectious Diseases 19
 2.2.3 The Impact of Technology on Climate Change and Infectious Diseases 20
2.3 Dynamics of Climate Change on Specific Infectious Diseases 21
 2.3.1 Climate Change and COVID-19 21
 2.3.2 Climate Change and the Hendra Virus 22
 2.3.3 Climate Change and the Influenza Virus 22
 2.3.4 Climate Change and Cholera 23
2.4 The Usefulness of the One Health Approach to Combat Climate Change-Dependent Pandemics 25
2.5 Conclusion 26
References 26

2.1 INTRODUCTION

Since the 16th century, when the term *pandemic* was first used to describe the continuous spread of a disease in a country (Kelly, 2011; Piret and Boivin, 2021), there have been recorded processions of pandemics that each shaped human history and society, including the very basic principles of modern medicine and health sciences (Huremović, 2019). Throughout history, catastrophic pandemics have posed a severe threat to sustaining life. While some of these events may have happened centuries or even decades apart, they have occurred in tandem and at global scales that have become increasingly common in recent years. As a result, different regions of the world have recorded one or more pandemics at different times and conditions

DOI: 10.1201/9781003288732-2

(Piret and Boivin, 2021). In addition, humanity has previously been afflicted by 'major pandemics and epidemics such as plague, cholera, flu, severe acute respiratory syndrome coronavirus (SARS-CoV) and Middle East respiratory syndrome coronavirus (MERS-CoV)' (Piret and Boivin, 2021). Within the last two decades, before the COVID-19 pandemic (2019), there have been at least five known epidemics or 'near pandemics' and pandemics around the globe: namely, the severe acute respiratory syndrome (SARS) (2003), influenza (2009), chikungunya (2014), and Zika (2015) (Morens et al., 2020). While pandemics might have previously been attributed to God's wrath against humanity (Jones, 2003), or political manipulations (Burkle, 2020), advances in research have implicated climate change as a driving factor in the occurrence of pandemics or infectious diseases alongside other interactions between humans and the environment (Colwell, 1998; Epstein, 2001; Flahault et al., 2016; Greer et al., 2008; Patz et al., 1878; Shuman, 2010, 2011).

2.2 CLIMATE CHANGE FACTORS ENHANCING INFECTIOUS DISEASE RATE

Climate change is any change occurring to the planet's climate that is either permanent or lasting for a long period. Climate change, alone or in combination with other environmental, social, and political variables, has evolved to make infections more transmissible. Because of the disturbance of biodiversity, which disrupts socio-ecological systems and brings people, vectors, animals, and diseases into closer contact, over 60% of human illnesses are zoonotic (Fornace et al., 2019). In Africa, climatic phenomena like El Niño and La Niña have been linked to a rise in arboviral, mosquito-borne diseases such as Rift Valley fever, cholera, malaria, and chikungunya. In contrast, drought in Northeast Brazil and Southeast Asia has been linked to increased dengue, Zika, and yellow fever, not excluding most 20th-century pandemics like seasonal influenza in Europe and the Americas, which have been statistically correlated with the La Niña phenomenon (Flahault et al., 2016).

2.2.1 Anthropogenic Factors of Climate Change and Infectious Diseases

Anthropogenic climate change factors refer to human impact on the earth's climate. However, due to the intricate interaction between global, regional, and local dynamics, it is challenging to ascribe climate change only to natural impacts or to the greenhouse effect of carbon dioxide, methane, and other greenhouse gases, which rapidly accumulate in the atmosphere due to burning fossil fuels and other human activities (Engels, 2016). Independently, anthropogenic global warming is predicted to cause premature death through rising seas, dry areas, severe storms, and heatwaves (Parncutt, 2019); this outcome could be devastating in terms of pandemic outcomes.

For example, the biodiversity of some mammals, such as bats, is a culprit in most pandemics due to habitat destruction by human activities. In addition, climate change has been implicated as a significant driver of infectious diseases. In a situation of environmental change due to human activity, animals like bats, with basal heat-shock protein expression and the loss of the interferon-inducible protein 20X/16 (PYHIN) protein family (Lorentzen et al., 2020), remain effective zoonotic causes of infectious diseases or pandemics.

2.2.2 Demographic Factors of Climate Change and Infectious Diseases

Several demographic factors contributing to climate change, such as urbanisation, population growth, land use change, migration, ageing, and changing birth rates, are related drivers of the transmission of infectious diseases and outbreaks. 'Urbanisation is the result of migration from rural to urban locales and the imbalance between death and fertility rates in urban and rural locales.' The effects of urbanisation, such as environmental contaminants, negatively impact health (Reyes et al., 2013), since cities may become incubators where all of the conditions are fulfilled for epidemics to emerge (Loutan, 2012). For example, increased shared airspace increases exposure to the influenza virus in areas of high population density. Deteriorating sanitation and hygiene and increased water pollution due to urbanisation contribute to outbreaks of diseases such as cholera. The ozone layer is affected by pollutant emissions, resulting in either warming or cooling effects on the earth. This promotes favourable conditions for opportunistic pathogens or their reservoirs, resulting in outbreaks, epidemics, or pandemics (Campbell-Lendrum and Corvalán, 2007; Jung et al., 2018; US EPA, 2014).

Biodiversity and climate change are interconnected, with biodiversity affected by climate change, negatively impacting human well-being (Hansen et al., 2012; Marques et al., 2019). Degradation of ecosystems and the loss of species variety puts the whole ecosystem at risk, increasing the likelihood of infectious disease outbreaks and other adverse health impacts on both people and animals. For example, the cases of Ebola virus disease, avian influenza (H5N1, H7N9), and H1N1 virus disease might have evolved from deforestation and habitat encroachment, which increased breeding sites and vectors, migration of susceptible people, and increased contact and pathogen transmission among captive birds, wild birds, and people (Malhi et al., 2020; Soh et al., 2019). In addition, when habitats are degraded, there are changes in species composition across the disturbance gradient. Resilient species are more likely to be generalists than threatened species and are hence adaptable to climatic change and likely to facilitate the transmission of opportunistic infectious agents, promoting outbreaks (Soh et al., 2019).

While ageing is a natural process, contemporary debates link climate change as a public health threat, particularly for the elderly, who are vulnerable to specific climate change consequences such as heatwaves (Frumkin et al., 2012). Older people experience physiological changes as part of the ageing process and are usually vulnerable and trapped in poor environments due to lack of mobility, disability, and increased risk of heat-related illnesses (Harper, 2019). Moreover, with less effective immune systems, the elderly may serve as a reservoir of infectious disease agents, as their systems present possible conditions for pathogens to mutate. For example, high ambient temperatures have been found to dampen adaptive immunity to influenza A virus infection (Moriyama and Ichinohe, 2019). In addition, recent evidence shows that overheating the body beyond 38 °C, either through physical exercise or directly due to environmental heatwaves, has detrimental effects on the performance of the innate immune system (Presbitero et al., 2021; Ramírez Otarola et al., 2018). This might suggest that climate change makes humans more susceptible to opportunistic disease agents.

2.2.3 The Impact of Technology on Climate Change and Infectious Diseases

It is undeniable that technology and climate change have an existing complex relationship. Technological advances in the 20th century have evolved with several advantages against climate change, including, but not limited to, reduced carbon emissions, reduced energy consumption, producing cleaner energy, and ensuring an eco-friendly agricultural system (Chen et al., 2020).

While existing evidence has positively emphasised that technological advances have contributed to reducing carbon emissions, little emphasis has been given to the indirect impact of technological progress on economic growth, which leads to changes in carbon dioxide emissions due to excessive consumption of energy (Li and Wang, 2017). Li and Wang observed that while technology did indeed cut aggregate carbon dioxide emissions, the beneficial effects of technological advancement on carbon dioxide emissions may have been overstated relative to the adverse effects. The significance of new technology in combating global climate change is determined by its inherent advantages and ability to produce energy at a lower cost than fossil fuels and the dangers of overuse.

On the other hand, some new threats from infectious diseases do not come from changes in the microorganisms themselves. Human activities can contribute to these by providing innovative, evolutionary improvements that might risk the community. In most situations, benefits are unknowingly offered as a by-product of technology in health or other sectors (Breiman, 1996). For example, a current debate revolves around the possibility that technology might contribute to spreading infectious illnesses such as COVID-19 by using smart portable devices, such as smartphones. Excessive use of wireless devices has also been linked to reducing human immunity (Pall, 2018) and could increase vulnerability to both infectious and non-communicable illnesses.

Thus, technological development has direct repercussions on climate change, which provides a suitable setting for the spread of infectious disease agents. It has also been shown to have direct and indirect implications on putting people in a vulnerable condition to infectious disease transmission and infection. However, a halt to innovative development is neither a viable nor a desirable option for stopping health threats resulting from technology (Breiman, 1996) in view of the benefits brought about by technology, such as (1) predicting disease risk and ensuring preparedness through artificial intelligence technology, (2) preventing spread through reliable, real-time data and analytics, and (3) saving lives through enabling technologies, e.g., 5G technologies (Ahmad, 2020).

2.3 DYNAMICS OF CLIMATE CHANGE ON SPECIFIC INFECTIOUS DISEASES

Environmental factors like temperature, rainfall, and humidity, impacted by climate change, significantly contribute to many infectious diseases (Tong et al., 2021). Disease spread is observed in conditions of increased climate variability and a decreased diurnal temperature range (DTR), permitting infectious agents to adapt faster than the hosts, grow, and spread further. According to specific reports, DTR has been shown to modify processes such as development compared with similar constant mean temperatures, making transmission viable at lower mean temperatures and perhaps preventing transmission at higher mean temperatures (Rohr and Cohen, 2020). Climate variability has also been linked to increased direct transmission of illnesses in wildlife. The thermal mismatch hypothesis attempts to explain how changing temperatures impact infection outcomes in that 'as environmental conditions shift away from those typically experienced by parasites (the infectious agent) and hosts (but remain within the threshold density of hosts), parasites often outperform hosts.' Hence, parasites thrive in nature at temperatures where they dominate the host rather than at temperatures where they thrive in isolation (Moriyama and Ichinohe, 2019; Rohr and Cohen, 2020).

A broad array of terrestrial, aquatic, nearshore, and estuarine systems, and systems outside the purview of biology, influence how climate change can affect infectious diseases. However, temperature and precipitation are often critical environmental drivers of infectious disease, including waterborne diseases like cholera, malaria, parasitic helminths, and fungal infections, which could alter disease dynamics and promote or exacerbate outbreaks in humans and wildlife (Rohr and Cohen, 2020; Thomas, 2020).

2.3.1 Climate Change and COVID-19

Before the COVID-19 pandemic, the climate change dilemma was perceived to be the most severe challenge that humanity might ever face. However, the parallels between climate change and COVID-19 sparked debate about which caused or influenced which. While some suggest that climate change may have triggered the COVID-19 outbreak, others contend that it did not. For example, during the COVID-19 phases, some private enterprises boosted waste and pollutant output because of the high usage of plastics and personal vehicles, which may have influenced climatic variability (Loureiro and Alló, 2021). Although scientists denied, based on visual inspection, that COVID-19 is less prevalent in regions closer to the equator where heat and humidity are high, there has been evidence indicating that climate change had a part in COVID-19's rise. For example, Chen et al. (2021) reported that 'a country, which is located 1,000 km closer to the equator, could expect 33% fewer cases per million inhabitants' and attributed this observation to the higher temperatures and intense UV radiation.

2.3.2 Climate Change and the Hendra Virus

The Hendra virus, whose vector is the pteropid bat, is classified as a biosafety level 4 organism (the same as Ebola virus) and emerging zoonotic pathogen. For example, the virus shows a spatio-temporal dynamic in Australia, with spikes in autumn and winter (a few cases, about 20%, occurring in spring and summer). It spreads to people by close contact with mares and foals and their bodily fluids, making disease transmission and epidemics more likely. In addition, virus dispersion by pteropid bats is more reliant on food supplies, such as nectar, pollen, and fruits, particularly those produced by eucalyptus trees in woodlands and open forests, which are influenced by seasonal climate triggers (e.g., regular temperature changes) (Yuen et al., 2021).

2.3.3 Climate Change and the Influenza Virus

Influenza or flu is an acute respiratory viral disease characterised by a sudden fever, headache, body ache, fatigue, general vertigo, and dry cough, with possible complications like long-lasting heart or lung diseases, metabolic syndromes like diabetes, and immune-related disorders, especially in the elderly (Blümel et al., 2009; Goodwins et al., 2019). Humanity experienced three influenza pandemics by the 21st century, all caused by different subtypes of influenza virus A, including H1N1 (1918), H2N2 (1957), and H3N2 (1968), and influenza A (H1N1) pdm09 virus (2009) (Garten et al., 2009; Kilbourne, 2006). These pandemics significantly impacted global mortality and morbidity with a tremendous financial burden.

A systematic review on the impact of climate change and influenza analysed 50 scientific papers that met the inclusion criteria. The authors conclude that none of the studies included in their review showed a direct link between flu and climate change (Goodwins et al., 2019). Despite this, numerous studies have shown a link between influenza and seasonality or weather conditions. For example, using a simulation model, a study showed a significant association between influenza propagation and humidity and temperature (Singh et al., 2020). The study observed a 1.6% increase in infection rate with a 10% drop in relative humidity, while an estimated 1.1% decrease in infection rate was associated with every 1-degree temperature rise. A scoping review showed a similar trend between influenza and temperature, revealing an inverse relationship whereby lower temperatures were linked to higher disease incidence (Lane et al., 2022a).

Furthermore, Towers et al. (2013) looked at the likelihood of increasing winter seasons on the incidence of influenza in the USA. The authors examined data from 1997 to 1998 and from 2012 to 2013. They observed that warmer winters preceded severe epidemics with early onset. They therefore suggested that fewer people were infected with influenza during warm winters. However, they warned that a significantly large susceptible population would go into the following season, leading to early and severe epidemics, and that this could be exacerbated by continued global warming. Despite these observations, a study in Australia found that irregular temperature and humidity variations could not predict local influenza epidemic onset timings (Lam et al., 2020).

These discrepancies in association between climate change and influenza indicate that other factors such as urbanisation, changing land use and population density could be involved, thus requiring further studies to prepare for any potential future outbreak (Lane et al., 2022b). Therefore, continuous evaluation and revision of risk assessment and pandemic preparedness measures must include information from such studies globally (Harrington et al., 2021).

2.3.4 Climate Change and Cholera

Cholera, an acute diarrhoeal disease caused by the bacterium *Vibrio cholerae*, affects between 3 and 5 million people, leading to up to 143,000 deaths, yearly worldwide (WHO, 2022). *V. cholerae* is primarily found in waters with high salt content (Vezzulli et al., 2010), although the organism has also adapted to surviving and thriving in freshwater milieus (Abia et al., 2016; Daboul et al., 2020). Thus, this pathogen's main transmission route is through consuming contaminated water or foods (Patel et al., 2009; Traore et al., 2012).

Several environmental factors influence the survival of this pathogen and hence, its transmission from these environmental sources to humans (Vezzulli et al., 2010). Thus, cholera transmission and outbreaks have been associated with climate change, impacting numerous environmental parameters such as temperature, floods, and droughts. The relation between cholera outbreaks and the environment cannot be overemphasised, as this has been reviewed extensively by many authors worldwide (Asadgol et al., 2020; Christaki et al., 2020; Lipp et al., 2002; De Magny et al., 2008; Rodó et al., 2002). For example, cholera outbreaks were correlated with rising sea surface temperature and flooding following prolonged monsoon rains in Bangladesh (Patz and Olson, 2006; Rodó et al., 2002). Similarly, in a narrative review by Christaki et al. (2020), the authors summarised that sea surface temperature and carbon dioxide and oxygen concentrations increased sea pollution, which altered seawater pH and salt levels, affecting the pathogen's replication, while sea-level rise, rainfall, floods, and droughts influenced the spread of disease. In another review, the authors observed through a literature search that cholera cases showed distinct seasonal patterns in endemic areas, with cases increasing during warmer climates; higher temperatures affect zooplankton blooms, which are a significant reservoir of *V. cholerae* in the aquatic environment (Lipp et al., 2002). The authors further stipulated that changing climatic conditions could have influenced the emergence of novel toxigenic strains, since even in endemic areas, the O1 strain (most associated with outbreaks) was less often isolated from the environment than the non-O1 strains.

Furthermore, natural events like droughts and floods associated with climate change would affect water quality and quantity, thus adversely impacting sanitation conditions and increasing human exposure and vulnerability to cholera (Asadgol et al., 2020). Drought, for example, causes migration of populations and refugee movements, leading to the continuous spread of the disease. This scenario has been experienced in Mozambique, Zimbabwe, and the Democratic Republic of Congo (DRC) (Charnley et al., 2022). Here, the authors report that the 1991–1992 drought in Mozambique led to massive population migration into Zimbabwe, leading to a fast-spreading cholera outbreak in the two countries. Similarly, the 1994 Rwandan genocide forced people into the DRC, resulting in a similar disease spread.

Using an artificial neural network, a study in Iran simulated the potential impact of climate change on cholera outbreaks. In this study, the authors observed a seasonal trend in the occurrence and spread of the infection and anticipated that cholera cases would increase by 2050 due to warmer and wetter weather conditions. They also observed that cholera was strongly correlated with rainfall, concluding that higher temperatures and increased rain favoured *V. cholerae*'s replication (Asadgol et al., 2019).

The impact of climate change on some environmental factors and how they subsequently affect the outbreak and spread of cholera is represented in Figure 2.1.

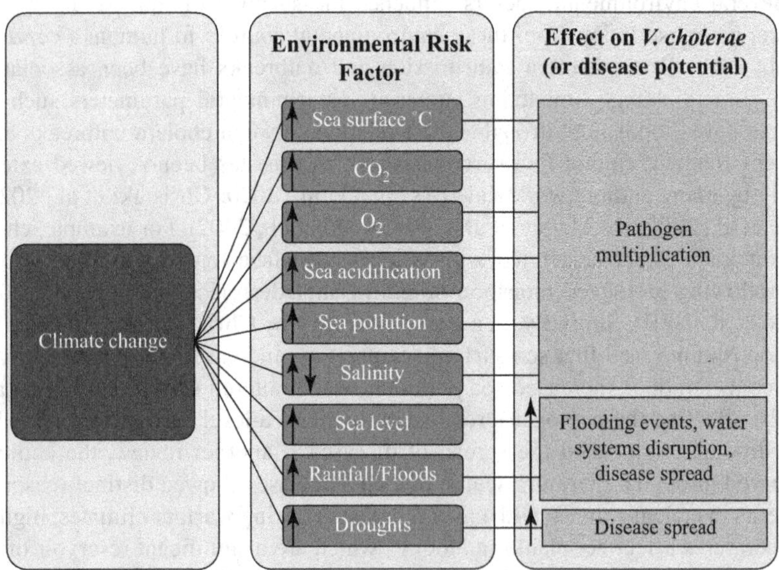

FIGURE 2.1 Effect of climate change on environmental factors and impact on cholera disease. The arrows indicate an increased (upward) or decreased (downward) trend. Salinity may rise or fall depending on increasing or decreasing rainfall (Christaki et al., 2020).

2.4 THE USEFULNESS OF THE ONE HEALTH APPROACH TO COMBAT CLIMATE CHANGE-DEPENDENT PANDEMICS

It has been demonstrated that human health is closely linked to animal and environmental health. The implication is that any intervention to address human health must consider the animals and the environment in which these humans and animals reside. Therefore, the World Health Organization and other international bodies have advocated for a One Health approach to tackling human diseases (Dukoska et al., 2010). This concept calls for effective multisectoral communication between human, animal, and environmental health (including plants) (Destoumieux-Garzon et al., 2018). From this perspective, approaching the fight against disease would ensure that more efficient and sustainable outcomes are achieved. In addition, this would further ensure that all potential reservoirs were identified and adequately addressed. Indeed, the One Health concept is needed if any fight against pandemics is to be won.

For example, after the first COVID-19 infection case in China in November 2019, scientists sought to understand the source of the virus. Investigation at the Wuhan market identified genetic material of the SARS-CoV-2 virus in human and environmental samples, making the market the epicentre for the disease (Maxmen, 2022). Many other studies later speculated that the virus must have jumped host from bats or pangolins into humans (Dhama et al., 2020; Mallapaty, 2021; Voskarides, 2022). Despite this realisation, measures to fight the pandemic were limited to restricting human-to-human contact by imposing social distancing, hand sanitisation, wearing masks, and banning travel. Finally, however, more scientific evidence emerged, reporting the extended survival of the viral particle on surfaces (Gonçalves et al., 2021; Liu et al., 2021; Marzoli et al., 2021; Riddell et al., 2020).

Another link between the virus and the environment emerged after it was reported that diarrhoea was one of the symptoms of COVID-19 and that the virus could be shed in the faeces of patients and asymptomatic carriers (Liu et al., 2021). This discovery spurred the shift to wastewater-based epidemiology to understand the spread of the infection within communities (Maida et al., 2022; Monteiro et al., 2022; Prado et al., 2021; Sanjuán and Domingo-Calap, 2021). Thus, several studies have looked at the environmental factors favouring the spread of COVID-19. For example, it was reported that temperature, air moisture, ultraviolet rays, and extreme weather conditions could influence the risk of infection with and the severity of COVID-19, as these factors could affect the host's immunity, the environmental survival of the virus, and human movement and behaviours (Weaver et al., 2022). Another study evaluated the mortality rate and severity of COVID-19 in Europe and concluded that these two parameters were significantly influenced by seasonality. As with other infectious diseases, several other authors have reported links between environmental factors and COVID-19 (Azuma et al., 2020; Kong et al., 2021; Sanchez-Piedra et al., 2022).

Therefore, these studies show the role of animals and the environment in the outbreak and severity of human diseases, some of which led to global pandemics.

The studies' findings highlight the importance of approaching pandemics from a One Health perspective. Any attempt to address the diseases in one sector of the triad, ignoring the other sectors, would be erroneous. However, studies that promptly evaluated the potential role of humans, animals, and the environment would identify hotspots and potential reservoirs, allowing effective and swift preventive measures to be implemented.

2.5 CONCLUSION

Infectious diseases have been part of human history and continue to be experienced today. Therefore, disease outbreaks are almost inevitable, and future events will still occur. Changing climatic conditions affect environmental factors that have an impact on pathogens' ecology and behaviour. These environmental factors also affect human migration, behaviour, and immunity. It is evident that climate change has influenced past and present pandemics and will affect the emergence of future ones. However, while climate change has been apparent in some cases, like cholera, this has not been the case with other pandemics, like influenza. This calls for further studies focusing on the interplay of these factors and their relation to pathogens and human health. Nevertheless, achieving success against or preventing future pandemics will require a One Health approach.

REFERENCES

Abia, A. L. K., Ubomba-Jaswa, E., and Momba, M. N. B. (2016). Prevalence of pathogenic microorganisms and their correlation with the abundance of indicator organisms in riverbed sediments. *Int. J. Environ. Sci. Technol.* 13(12), 2905–2916. doi:10.1007/s13762-016-1116-y.

Ahmad, F. (2020). Forbes: How technology can help combat the spread of disease. *Forbes*. Available at: https://www.forbes.com/sites/forbesbusinesscouncil/2020/03/17/how-technology-can-help-combat-the-spread-of-disease/.

Asadgol, Z., Badirzadeh, A., Niazi, S., Mokhayeri, Y., Kermani, M., Mohammadi, H., and Gholami, M. (2020). How climate change can affect cholera incidence and prevalence? A systematic review. *Environ. Sci. Pollut. Res. Int.* 27(28), 34906–34926. doi:10.1007/s11356-020-09992-7.

Asadgol, Z., Mohammadi, H., Kermani, M., Badirzadeh, A., and Gholami, M. (2019). The effect of climate change on cholera disease: The road ahead using artificial neural network. *Plos One* 14(11), 1–20. doi:10.1371/journal.pone.0224813.

Azuma, K., Yanagi, U., Kagi, N., Kim, H., Ogata, M., and Hayashi, M. (2020). Environmental factors involved in SARS-CoV-2 transmission: Effect and role of indoor environmental quality in the strategy for COVID-19 infection control. *Environ. Health Prev. Med.* 25(1), 1–16. doi:10.1186/s12199-020-00904-2.

Blümel, J., Burger, R., Drosten, C., Gröner, A., Gürtler, L., Heiden, M., et al. (2009). Influenza virus. *Transfus. Med. Hemother.* 36(1), 32–39. doi:10.1159/000197314.

Breiman, R. F. (1996). Impact of technology on the emergence of infectious diseases. *Epidemiol. Rev.* 18(1), 4–9. doi:10.1093/oxfordjournals.epirev.a017915.

Burkle, F. M. (2020). Political intrusions into the international health regulations treaty and its impact on management of rapidly emerging zoonotic pandemics: What history tells us. *Prehosp. Disaster Med.* 35(4), 426–430. doi:10.1017/S1049023X20000515.

Campbell-Lendrum, D., and Corvalán, C. (2007). Climate change and developing-country cities: Implications for environmental health and equity. *J. Urban Heal.* 84(Supplement), 109–117. doi:10.1007/s11524-007-9170-x.

Charnley, G. E. C., Kelman, I., and Murray, K. A. (2022). Drought-related cholera outbreaks in Africa and the implications for climate change: A narrative review. *Pathog. Glob. Health* 116(1), 3–12. doi:10.1080/20477724.2021.1981716.

Chen, J., Gao, M., Mangla, S. K., Song, M., and Wen, J. (2020). Effects of technological changes on China's carbon emissions. *Technol. Forecast. Soc. Change* 153, 119938. doi:10.1016/j.techfore.2020.119938.

Chen, S., Prettner, K., Kuhn, M., Geldsetzer, P., Wang, C., Bärnighausen, T., and Bloom, D. E. (2021). Climate and the spread of COVID-19. *Sci. Rep.* 11(1), 9042. doi:10.1038/s41598-021-87692-z.

Christaki, E., Dimitriou, P., Pantavou, K., and Nikolopoulos, G. K. (2020). The impact of climate change on cholera: A review on the global status and future challenges. *Atmosphere (Basel)* 11(5), 1–11. doi:10.3390/ATMOS11050449.

Colwell, R., Epstein, P., Gubler, D., Hall, M., Reiter, P., Shukla, J., et al. (1998). Global climate change and infectious diseases. *Emerg. Infect. Dis.* 4(3), 451–452. doi:10.3201/eid0403.980327.

Daboul, J., Weghorst, L., DeAngelis, C., Plecha, S. C., Saul-McBeth, J., and Matson, J. S. (2020). Characterization of Vibrio cholerae isolates from freshwater sources in northwest Ohio. *Plos One* 15(9), 1–12. doi:10.1371/journal.pone.0238438.

Destoumieux-Garzon, D., Mavingui, P., Boetsch, G., Boissier, J., Darriet, F., Duboz, P., et al. (2018). The one health concept: 10 years old and a long road ahead. *Front. Vet. Sci.* 5, 14. doi:10.3389/fvets.2018.00014.

Dhama, K., Patel, S. K., Sharun, K., Pathak, M., Tiwari, R., Yatoo, M. I., et al. (2020). SARS-CoV-2 jumping the species barrier: Zoonotic lessons from SARS, MERS and recent advances to combat this pandemic virus. *Travel Med. Infect. Dis.* 37, 101830. doi:10.1016/j.tmaid.2020.101830.

Dukoska, V., Cvetkovik, I., Cvetkovik, A., and Hristovski, M. (2010). Concept of one health - A new professional imperative. *Maced. J. Med. Sci.* 3(3), 229–232. doi:10.3889/mjms.1857-5773.2010.0131.

Engels, A. (2016). Anthropogenic climate change: How to understand the weak links between scientific evidence, public perception, and low-carbon practices. *Energy Emiss Control. Technol.* 4, 17–26. doi:10.2147/EECT.S63005.

Epstein, P. R. (2001). Climate change and emerging infectious diseases. *Microbes Infect.* 3(9), 747–754. doi:10.1016/S1286-4579(01)01429-0.

Flahault, A., de Castaneda, R. R., and Bolon, I. (2016). Climate change and infectious diseases. *Public Health Rev.* 37(21). doi:10.1186/s40985-016-0035-2.

Fornace, K. M., Brock, P. M., Abidin, T. R., Grignard, L., Herman, L. S., Chua, T. H., et al. (2019). Environmental risk factors and exposure to the zoonotic malaria parasite *Plasmodium knowlesi* across northern Sabah, Malaysia: A population-based cross-sectional survey. *Lancet Planet. Heal.* 3(4), e179–e186. doi:10.1016/S2542-5196(19)30045-2.

Frumkin, H., Fried, L., and Moody, R. (2012). Aging, climate change, and legacy thinking. *Am. J. Public Health* 102(8), 1434–1438. doi:10.2105/AJPH.2012.300663.

Garten, R. J., Davis, C. T., Russell, C. A., Shu, B., Lindstrom, S., Balish, A., et al. (2009). Antigenic and genetic characteristics of swine-origin 2009 A(H1N1) influenza viruses circulating in humans. *Science* 325(5937), 197–201. doi:10.1126/science.1176225.

Gonçalves, J., da Silva, P. G., Reis, L., Nascimento, M. S. J., Koritnik, T., Paragi, M., and Mesquita, J. R. (2021). Surface contamination with SARS-CoV-2: A systematic review. *Sci. Total Environ.* 798, 149231. doi:10.1016/j.scitotenv.2021.149231.

Goodwins, L., Menzies, B., Osborne, N., and Muscatello, D. (2019). Human seasonal influenza and climate change: A systematic review of the methods used to examine the relationship between meteorological variables and influenza. *Environ. Epidemiol.* 3, 137. doi:10.1097/01.EE9.0000607256.48033.53.

Greer, A., Ng, V., and Fisman, D. (2008). Climate change and infectious diseases in North America: The road ahead. *Can. Med. Assoc. J.* 178(6), 715–722. http://www.cmaj.ca/content/178/6/715.short. Accessed November 27, 2013.

Hansen, A. J., DeFries, R. S., Turner, W., and van der Meer, F. D. (2012). Land use change and biodiversity: A synthesis of rates and consequences during the period of satellite imagery. In *Land Change Science*, eds. G. Gutman, A. C. Janetos, C. O. Justice, E. F. Moran, J. F. Mustard, R. R. Rindfuss, et al. Dordrecht: Springer Netherlands, pp. 277–299. Available at: http://link.springer.com/10.1007/978-1-4020-2562-4_16.

Harper, S. (2019). The convergence of population ageing with climate change. *J. Popul. Ageing* 12(4), 401–403. doi:10.1007/s12062-019-09255-5.

Harrington, W. N., Kackos, C. M., and Webby, R. J. (2021). The evolution and future of influenza pandemic preparedness. *Exp. Mol. Med.* 53(5), 737–749. doi:10.1038/s12276-021-00603-0.

Huremović, D. (2019). Brief history of pandemics (pandemics throughout history). In *Psychiatry of Pandemics*, ed. D. Huremović. Springer Nature. doi:10.1007/978-3-030-15346-5.

Jones, D. S. (2003). Virgin soils revisited. *William Mary Q.* 60(4), 703–742.

Jung, S. J., Mehta, J. S., and Tong, L. (2018). Effects of environment pollution on the ocular surface. *Ocul. Surf.* 16(2), 198–205. doi:10.1016/j.jtos.2018.03.001.

Kelly, H. (2011). The classical definition of a pandemic is not elusive. *Bull. World Health Organ.* 89(7), 540–541. doi:10.2471/BLT.11.088815.

Kilbourne, E. D. (2006). Influenza pandemics of the 20th century. *Emerg. Infect. Dis.* 12(1), 9–14. doi:10.3201/eid1201.051254.

Kong, J. D., Tekwa, E. W., and Gignoux-Wolfsohn, S. A. (2021). Social, economic, and environmental factors influencing the basic reproduction number of COVID-19 across countries. *Plos One* 16(6), 1–17. doi:10.1371/journal.pone.0252373.

Lam, E. K. S., Morris, D. H., Hurt, A. C., Barr, I. G., and Russell, C. A. (2020). The impact of climate and antigenic evolution on seasonal influenza virus epidemics in Australia. *Nat. Commun.* 11(1). doi:10.1038/s41467-020-16545-6.

Lane, M. A., Walawender, M., Carter, J., Brownsword, E. A., Landay, T., Gillespie, T. R., et al. (2022a). Climate change and influenza: A scoping review. *J. Clim. Chang Heal.* 5, 100084. doi:10.1016/j.joclim.2021.100084.

Lane, M. A., Walawender, M., Carter, J., Brownsword, E. A., Landay, T., Gillespie, T. R., et al. (2022b). Climate change and influenza: A scoping review. *J. Clim. Chang Heal.* 5, 100084. doi:10.1016/j.joclim.2021.100084.

Li, M., and Wang, Q. (2017). Will technology advances alleviate climate change? Dual effects of technology change on aggregate carbon dioxide emissions. *Energy Sustain. Dev.* 41, 61–68. doi:10.1016/j.esd.2017.08.004.

Lipp, E. K., Huq, A., and Colwell, R. R. (2002). Effects of global climate on infectious disease: The cholera model. *Clin. Microbiol. Rev.* 15(4), 757–770. doi:10.1128/CMR.15.4.757-770.2002.

Liu, Y., Li, T., Deng, Y., Liu, S., Zhang, D., Li, H., et al. (2021). Stability of SARS-CoV-2 on environmental surfaces and in human excreta. *J. Hosp. Infect.* 107, 105–107. doi:10.1016/j.jhin.2020.10.021.

Lorentzen, H. F., Benfield, T., Stisen, S., and Rahbek, C. (2020). Covid-19 is possibly a consequence of the anthropogenic biodiversity crisis and climate changes. *Dan. Med. J.* 67(5).

Loureiro, M. L., and Alló, M. (2021). How has the COVID-19 pandemic affected the climate change debate on Twitter? *Environ. Sci. Policy* 124, 451–460. doi:10.1016/j.envsci.2021.07.011.

Loutan, L. (2012). Urbanization reshaping infectious diseases. *Int. J. Infect. Dis.* 16, e20. doi:10.1016/j.ijid.2012.05.053.

De Magny, G. C., Murtugudde, R., Sapiano, M. R. P., Nizam, A., Brown, C. W., Busalacchi, A. J., et al. (2008). Environmental signatures associated with cholera epidemics. *Proc. Natl. Acad. Sci. U. S. A.* 105(46), 17676–17681. doi:10.1073/pnas.0809654105.

Maida, C. M., Amodio, E., Mazzucco, W., La Rosa, G., Lucentini, L., Suffredini, E., et al. (2022). Wastewater-based epidemiology for early warning of SARS-COV-2 circulation: A pilot study conducted in Sicily, Italy. *Int. J. Hyg. Environ. Health* 242. doi:10.1016/j.ijheh.2022.113948.

Malhi, Y., Franklin, J., Seddon, N., Solan, M., Turner, M. G., Field, C. B., and Knowlton, N. (2020). Climate change and ecosystems: Threats, opportunities and solutions. *Philos. Trans. R. Soc. B Biol. Sci.* doi:10.1098/rstb.2019.0104.

Mallapaty, S. (2021). Did the coronavirus jump from animals to people twice? *Nature* 597(7877), 458–459. doi:10.1038/d41586-021-02519-1.

Marques, A., Martins, I. S., Kastner, T., Plutzar, C., Theurl, M. C., Eisenmenger, N., et al. (2019). Increasing impacts of land use on biodiversity and carbon sequestration driven by population and economic growth. *Nat. Ecol. Evol.* 3(4), 628–637. doi:10.1038/s41559-019-0824-3.

Marzoli, F., Bortolami, A., Pezzuto, A., Mazzetto, E., Piro, R., Terregino, C., et al. (2021). A systematic review of human coronaviruses survival on environmental surfaces. *Sci. Total Environ.* 778, 146191. doi:10.1016/j.scitotenv.2021.146191.

Maxmen, A. (2022). Wuhan market was epicentre of pandemib's start, study suggests. *Nature* 603(7899).

Monteiro, S., Rente, D., Cunha, M. V., Gomes, M. C., Marques, T. A., Lourenço, A. B., et al. (2022). A wastewater-based epidemiology tool for COVID-19 surveillance in Portugal. *Sci. Total Environ.* 804. doi:10.1016/j.scitotenv.2021.150264.

Morens, D. M., Daszak, P., and Taubenberger, J. K. (2020). Escaping Pandora's box — Another novel coronavirus. *N. Engl. J. Med.* 382(14), 1293–1295. doi:10.1056/nejmp2002106.

Moriyama, M., and Ichinohe, T. (2019). High ambient temperature dampens adaptive immune responses to influenza A virus infection. *Proc. Natl. Acad. Sci. U. S. A.* 116(8), 3118–3125. doi:10.1073/pnas.1815029116.

Pall, M. L. (2018). Wi-fi is an important threat to human health. *Environ. Res.* 164, 405–416. doi:10.1016/j.envres.2018.01.035.

Parncutt, R. (2019). The human cost of anthropogenic global warming: Semi-quantitative prediction and the 1,000-tonne rule. *Front. Psychol.* 10. Available at: https://www.frontiersin.org/article/10.3389/fpsyg.2019.02323.

Patel, N. M., Wong, M., Little, E., Ramos, A. X., Kolli, G., Fox, K. M., et al. (2009). Vibrio cholerae non-O1 infection in cirrhotics: Case report and literature review. *Transpl. Infect. Dis.* 11(1), 54–56. doi:10.1111/j.1399-3062.2008.00339.x.

Patz, J. A., Githeko, A. K., Mccarty, J. P., Hussein, S., and Confalonieri, U. (1878). Climate change and infectious diseases. 103–132.

Patz, J. A., and Olson, S. H. (2006). Climate change and health: Global to local influences on disease risk. *Ann. Trop. Med. Parasitol.* 100(5–6), 535–549. doi:10.1179/136485906X97426.

Piret, J., and Boivin, G. (2021). Pandemics throughout history. *Front. Microbiol.* 11. doi:10.3389/fmicb.2020.631736.

Prado, T., Fumian, T. M., Mannarino, C. F., Resende, P. C., Motta, F. C., Eppinghaus, A. L. F., et al. (2021). Wastewater-based epidemiology as a useful tool to track SARS-CoV-2 and support public health policies at municipal level in Brazil. *Water Res.* 191, 116810. doi:10.1016/j.watres.2021.116810.

Presbitero, A., Melnikov, V. R., Krzhizhanovskaya, V. V., and Sloot, P. M. A. (2021). A unifying model to estimate the effect of heat stress in the human innate immunity during physical activities. *Sci. Rep.* 11(1), 1–18. doi:10.1038/s41598-021-96191-0.

Ramírez Otarola, N., Espinoza, J., Kalergis, A. M., and Sabat Kirkwood, A. P. (2018). Is there an effect of environmental temperature on the response to an antigen and the metabolic rate in pups of the rodent *Octodon degus*? *J. Therm. Biol.* doi:10.1016/j.jtherbio.2017.10.005.

Reyes, R., Ahn, R., Thurber, K., and Burke, T. F. (2013). Urbanization and infectious diseases: General principles, historical perspectives, and contemporary challenges. In *Challenges in Infectious Diseases*, ed. I. W. Fong. New York: Springer, pp. 123–146. doi:10.1007/978-1-4614-4496-1_4.

Riddell, S., Goldie, S., Hill, A., Eagles, D., and Drew, T. W. (2020). The effect of temperature on persistence of SARS-CoV-2 on common surfaces. *Virol. J.* 17(1), 1–7. doi:10.1186/s12985-020-01418-7.

Rodó, X., Pascual, M., Fuchs, G., and Faruque, A. S. G. (2002). ENSO and cholera: A nonstationary link related to climate change? *Proc. Natl. Acad. Sci. U. S. A.* 99(20), 12901–12906. doi:10.1073/pnas.182203999.

Rohr, J. R., and Cohen, J. M. (2020). Understanding how temperature shifts could impact infectious disease. *Plos Biol.* 18(11), e3000938. doi:10.1371/journal.pbio.3000938.

Sanchez-Piedra, C., Gamiño-Arroyo, A.-E., Cruz-Cruz, C., and Prado-Galbarro, F.-J. (2022). Impact of environmental and individual factors on COVID-19 mortality in children and adolescents in Mexico: An observational study. *Lancet Reg. Heal. Am.* 8, 100184. doi:10.1016/j.lana.2022.100184.

Sanjuán, R., and Domingo-Calap, P. (2021). Reliability of wastewater analysis for monitoring COVID-19 incidence revealed by a long-term follow-up study. *Front. Virol.* 1, 1–9. doi:10.3389/fviro.2021.776998.

Shuman, E. K. (2010). Global climate change and infectious diseases. *N. Engl. J. Med.* 362(12), 1061–1063. doi:10.3201/eid0403.980327.

Shuman, E. K. (2011). Global climate change and infectious diseases. *Int. J. Occup. Environ. Med.* 2(1), 11–19. Available at: http://www.ncbi.nlm.nih.gov/pubmed/23022814.

Singh, D. E., Marinescu, M. C., Carretero, J., Delgado-Sanz, C., Gomez-Barroso, D., and Larrauri, A. (2020). Evaluating the impact of the weather conditions on the influenza propagation. *BMC Infect. Dis.* 20(1), 1–14. doi:10.1186/s12879-020-04977-w.

Soh, M. C. K., Mitchell, N. J., Ridley, A. R., Butler, C. W., Puan, C. L., and Peh, K. S.-H. (2019). Impacts of habitat degradation on tropical montane biodiversity and ecosystem services: A systematic map for identifying future research priorities. *Front. For. Glob. Chang.* 2. Available at: https://www.frontiersin.org/article/10.3389/ffgc.2019.00083.

Thomas, M. B. (2020). Epidemics on the move: Climate change and infectious disease. *Plos Biol.* 18(11), e3001013. doi:10.1371/journal.pbio.3001013.

Tong, S., Ebi, K., and Olsen, J. (2021). Infectious disease, the climate, and the future. *Environ. Epidemiol.* 5(2), e133. doi:10.1097/EE9.0000000000000133.

Towers, S., Chowell, G., Hameed, R., Jastrebski, M., Khan, M., Meeks, J., et al. (2013). Climate change and influenza: The likelihood of early and severe influenza seasons following warmer than average winters. *Plos Curr.* 5. doi:10.1371/currents.flu.3679b56a3a5313dc7c043fb944c6f138.

Traore, S. G., Bonfoh, B., Krabi, R., Odermatt, P., Utzinger, J., Rose, K. N., et al. (2012). Risk of Vibrio transmission linked to the consumption of crustaceans in coastal towns of Cote d'Ivoire. *J. Food Prot.* 75(6), 1004–1011. doi:10.4315/0362-028X.JFP-11-472.

US EPA, O. R. D. (2014). *Air Quality and Climate Change Research.* Available at: https://www.epa.gov/air-research/air-quality-and-climate-change-research.

Vezzulli, L., Pruzzo, C., Huq, A., and Colwell, R. R. (2010). Environmental reservoirs of Vibrio cholerae and their role in cholera. *Environ. Microbiol. Rep.* 2(1), 27–33. doi:10.1111/j.1758-2229.2009.00128.x.

Voskarides, K. (2022). SARS-CoV-2: Tracing the origin, tracking the evolution. *BMC Med. Genomics* 15(1), 1–5. doi:10.1186/s12920-022-01208-w.

Weaver, A. K., Head, J. R., Gould, C. F., Carlton, E. J., and Remais, J. V. (2022). Environmental factors influencing COVID-19 incidence and severity. *Annu. Rev. Public Health* 43, 271–291. doi:10.1146/annurev-publhealth-052120-101420.

WHO. (2022). Supporting cholera outbreak response. Available at: https://www.who.int/activities/supporting-cholera-outbreak-response.

Yuen, K. Y., Fraser, N. S., Henning, J., Halpin, K., Gibson, J. S., Betzien, L., and Stewart, A. J. (2021). Hendra virus: Epidemiology dynamics in relation to climate change, diagnostic tests and control measures. *One Heal.* 12, 100207. doi:10.1016/j.onehlt.2020.100207.

3 Economic Outcomes of Emerging Pandemics and Their Implications for the Environment

Denis Nfor Yuni and Lehlohonolo Mantsi

CONTENTS

3.1 Introduction 33
3.2 Economic Implications for Economic Growth and Financial Flows 34
3.3 Economic Effect on Global Value Chains 35
3.4 Economic Effect on ICT Development and Its Implications for the Environment 37
3.5 Economic Effect on Tourism and Travel 38
3.6 Opportunity Cost of the Fight Against Climate Change 39
3.7 Conclusion 41
References 42

3.1 INTRODUCTION

Twenty-first-century pandemics such as the 2003 SARS and COVID-19 have unique economic implications because of the way they are transmitted, similar to the 1889 Russian flu, the 1918 Spanish flu, and the 1957 Asian flu. The 1981 HIV/AIDS pandemic spread through blood and genital fluid, so it had different dynamics in terms of economic implications. The SARS and COVID-19 pandemics led to the implementation of travel bans; city, regional, and country lockdowns; and the lockdown of non-essential businesses. These affected economic activities in general, directly affecting macroeconomic indicators such as inflation, financial flows, international trade, investments, exchange rates, and economic growth. The tourism, manufacturing, and service (especially transportation, hospitality, and retail) industry, in general, witnessed massive economic shocks due to the management of these pandemics.

The economic implications of emerging pandemics can be classified as direct or indirect. The indirect implications, in most cases, turned out to be more far-reaching. These financial consequences of the pandemics had varying effects on the environment. Some are already being witnessed, such as the dwindling

DOI: 10.1201/9781003288732-3

commitment to climate financing, food waste, especially in 2020, and the inability to manage tourist sites like botanical gardens due to a fall in demand. Others will manifest in the medium and long term, such as the production of more electronics for information and communication technology (ICT) consumption, inefficient sources of fuelling electronic appliances, and the desire for production independence in some products due to the disruptions in global value chains (GVCs).

3.2 ECONOMIC IMPLICATIONS FOR ECONOMIC GROWTH AND FINANCIAL FLOWS

Emerging pandemics such as SARS and COVID-19 directly affected the economic environment of almost all economies. The restriction of movement directly affected production, consumption, markets, and supply chains, among others. SARS, which was predominant in Asia, fared relatively better. Nay and Shields (2019) reported that Hong Kong–China's supply chain was not affected by the restrictions during the SARS pandemic, and the cross-border movement of goods continued without significant disruption. Also, the rate of growth in the production of industrial goods as well as retail sales in China was relatively lower in May 2003, while the volume of exports remained stable throughout 2003, so the environment was not significantly affected.

Beyond China, Bio Enterprise Asia estimated the actual cost of health expenditure in East Asia linked to SARS at $50 billion, while the World Health Organization projected that the global cost of the SARS pandemic was about $30 billion towards the end of April 2003 (Roberts, 2003). Some estimates note that the economic effects in East Asia were only the compounding spillover effect of the global financial crisis, which was already on the way. However, it is essential to appreciate that the containment of SARS avoided further economic and environmental consequences.

COVID-19 had a broader and more significant economic effect than other recent pandemics due to its more extensive coverage and duration. The World Bank estimates that the world gross domestic product (GDP) growth rate in 2020 dropped by 3.29%, foreign direct investment (FDI) net inflows dropped by 0.019%, personal remittances dropped by 0.01%, and exports of goods and services as a percentage of GDP dropped by 0.06%. Of all the regions mentioned in this chapter, Europe and Central Asia had the lowest growth rate of –5.6% and FDI net inflows of −0.64; sub-Saharan Africa recorded the lowest growth rate in personal remittances of 0.14; and North America recorded the lowest growth rates in exports as a percentage of GDP of 0.14. It is worth noting that these regions recorded negative growth rates across most of the indicators. These figures may not represent the scientific impact of COVID-19 on these indicators, as control factors have not been regressed alongside; they infer that these economic indicators were negatively affected due to the massive restrictions caused by COVID-19 (Table 3.1).

TABLE 3.1
Key economic indicators growth rate between 2019 and 2020

Description	GDP (%)	FDI net inflows (%)	Personal remittances received (%)	Exports of goods and services as % of GDP
World	-3.29	–0.19	–0.01	–0.06
Arab World	-5.3	–0.02	0.03	-1.00
Europe and Central Asia	-5.6	–0.64	–0.06	–0.06
East Asia and the Pacific	–0.1	0.03	–0.02	–0.05
The Middle East and North Africa	–4	0.07	0.03	–
North America	-3.5	–0.32	–0.11	–0.14
Sub-Saharan Africa	-2	–0.05	–0.14	–0.13

Source: World Bank Indicators, 2022, https://data.worldbank.org/topic/economy-and-growth?view=chart.

These statistics point to the broader picture of the economic consequences of the COVID-19 restrictions. The fall in GDP in 2020 from 2019 could be connected to the fall in demand as restaurants and supermarkets were closed, the fall in production, and the closure of tourism and other recreational services. However, the fall in demand due to the closure of restaurants and supermarkets directly affected the environment, as it led to massive food wastage due to the interruption in supply chains and the perishable nature of some foods.

For example, by 4 April, 2020, *Wall Street Journal* reported that the closure of restaurants across the US had left cooks and large-scale farmers with tons of perishable food and meat to dispose of in haste; the *Guardian News* reported that billions of dollars were being wasted as producers moved from California and Florida due to highly perishable items. Similarly, an international study by Filho et al. (2021) documented an increase of about 43% and 53% in food waste and plastic packaging, respectively. It should be noted that this was unfortunate considering the number of persons going hungry in other parts of the world. More importantly, food wastage and consequent dumping is an environmental hazard that can cause groundwater pollution and contribute to global warming by emitting a natural by-product of the decomposition of organic material – landfill gas (made up of methane and carbon dioxide) (World Economic Forum, 2020).

3.3 ECONOMIC EFFECT ON GLOBAL VALUE CHAINS

GVCs refer to the interconnectedness of global businesses operated by numerous entities in various countries (Sturgeon and Memedović, 2011). Therefore, GVCs incorporate international transactions through cross-border trade, and this phenomenon has become an integral part of global economic development and relations. The Organisation for Economic Co-operation and Development (OECD) (2020) posits that COVID-19 affected GVCs in four key ways. The first is when firms involved in GVCs have some patients lose working days or die due to ill health. The other three reasons indirectly explain how COVID-19 affected GVCs: second, due to disruptions in the supply chain when production in one location is required as input for production further down the supply chain; third, referring to a demand shock where demand from different countries was turned down and could not be met; and lastly, the trade and investment policy risk, when governments tend to domesticate supply to ensure the sustainability of the supply.

The argument around GVCs rests on the efficiency in production and allocation of resources, reduced cost of production, division of labour and specialisation, and ultimately, substantial economic gains. External shocks posed by pandemics affect these gains from GVCs and most importantly, generate other disturbing economic concerns. Bonadio et al. (2020) showed that GVC disruptions resulting from COVID-19 were responsible for the loss of one-quarter of the GDP globally. Almost 80 countries executed export restrictions to safeguard critical commodities within their national borders, such as ventilators. The United States Institute for Supply Chain Management conducted a study in early 2020 to investigate how COVID-19-related export restrictions disrupted the GVC. Of 630 respondents, 599 indicated that the pandemic had negatively affected the GVC due to export ban strategies (Tripp, 2020).

The effect of the COVID-19 pandemic on GVCs was devastating because the pandemic started by hitting the factory of the world, China. Hence, the temporary shutting down of borders and transport limitations hampered the flow of exports and imports, so countries had to focus on import relief strategies (Matthes, 2020; Evenett, 2020). As a result, China, being the centre/foundation of several GVCs around the world, recorded a decrease of 4% in imports and 17% in exports, valued in US dollars, in January and February 2020 compared with the same period in 2019 (Seric et al., 2020). It is noteworthy that the majority of the goods that constitute imports are among products used as intermediates or raw materials in the production of other goods, such as textiles/fabrics and electrical and electronic equipment. Likewise, it is safe to infer that the same reason could be the source of the drop in exports.

The disruption of GVCs due to pandemics tends to stimulate countries to be self-sufficient. However, according to OECD (2021), interruptions in supply chains of critical, indispensable products as well as deficiencies of vital medicinal products in the heat of the COVID-19 pandemic have further demonstrated the interconnectedness between/among countries/regions via GVCs and re-ignited the debate on the risks and volatility associated with the alternative, which is the international disintegration of production units. Also, the United Nations Conference on Trade and Development (2020) opined that developing countries could consider consolidating some of the existing regional supply chains to diversify risk, decrease vulnerability, improve resilience, and promote manufacturing and industrial development by recognising and preserving horizontal and vertical linkages/associations and regional treaties/agreements. This will significantly enhance the growth of small firms, decrease transaction costs, and increase benefits from economies of scale.

As a result, countries are creating new production points, increasing the number of production plants globally. However, these production plants may be powered by inefficient climate sources, which increase carbon emissions and are unsuitable for the environment. On the flip side, this implies that major plants along GVCs that previously produced on a massive scale were forced to drastically reduce supply and even production capacity, leading to wastage of products and machinery, which is equally not good for the environment.

3.4 ECONOMIC EFFECT ON ICT DEVELOPMENT AND ITS IMPLICATIONS FOR THE ENVIRONMENT

The restrictions on physical meetings in closed and open spaces across the globe due to the pandemic led to an increment in ICT communication platforms. Work meetings, family meetings, association meetings, workshops, and conferences all had to be done online in almost all countries with varying lockdown measures. In addition, most daily work and reporting also had to be done on the internet to respect the lockdown measures. Thus, the use of internet services increased globally from 40% to 100% during the lockdown relative to pre-COVID lockdown levels; video-conferencing facilities like Zoom recorded a tenfold upsurge in usage by June 2020; content-delivery facilities like Akamai recorded a 30% upsurge in content usage in the same period; and cities like Bangalore recorded a 100% increase in internet traffic (Branscombe, 2020; De et al., 2020).

Shutting down schools and the 'Stay at Home' pandemic slogan increased the need to use televisions and computer gadgets such as phones and laptops. In May 2020, the use of cell phone services in the US showed that texting rose by 37%, social media use by 36%, shopping apps use by 23%, and video calling by 32% (Twigby, 2020). Oberoi and Singh (2020) postulate that even though the COVID-19 outbreak did not trigger Industry 5.0, it buttressed the reality of Industry 4.0, such that the use of and demand for robots, digital workflows, and automation are imminent.

On the other hand, Fortune Business Insights (2020) posited that the COVID-19 outbreak and its implications would likely reduce spending in the digital industry in 2020, thereby reducing the adoption of artificial intelligence (AI) solutions from 33.2% to 25.9% in 2020. Furthermore, before the COVID-19 pandemic, the AI retail market globally was projected to reach about $US4,075 million in 2020, but the outbreak reduced this projection to $US3,795 million by the end of 2020. Therefore, it is important to note that although ICT development funding declined generally, increased usage of ICT changed the dynamics of work and business structures, in most cases permanently. Thus, the increased ICT use is one of the few benefits of the COVID-19 pandemic.

Nevertheless, as much as we appreciate the ease in communication and all other benefits of using ICT, its implications for the environment are equally worth noting and worrisome. ICT contributes significant proportions of total carbon emissions globally due to its electricity use and the requisite cooling systems. It is estimated that ICT alone contributes about 10% of global energy and 4% of carbon emissions (ICTFOOTPRINT-EU, 2020). In addition, the production of phones and computer gadgets and waste from computer gadgets and accessories all contribute to more emissions and global warming. It is tempting to think that the massive increase in ICT usage is temporary, but the exposure of new users to different aspects of ICT and the benefits enjoyed by users will keep ICT demand significantly higher than it used to be. Therefore, there needs to be environmental awareness in ICT adoption as a mitigation mechanism for emerging pandemics such as COVID-19.

3.5 ECONOMIC EFFECT ON TOURISM AND TRAVEL

During pandemics like COVID-19 and SARS, some economic sectors are usually hit harder than others. For example, before the COVID-19 outbreak, tourism had become one of the most beneficial sectors of the world, contributing 10% of global GDP and above 320 million jobs worldwide (Behsudi, 2020). However, the United Nations World Trade Organization (2020) projected that revenues from the global tourism industry might drop by about US$910 billion to US$1.2 trillion in 2020, which could decrease global GDP by 1.5–2.8%. Meanwhile, Abbas et al. (2021) showed that global leisure and internal tourism declined to US$2.86 trillion, accounting for more than 50% loss in revenue. In addition, the US alone recorded a loss of more than US$297 billion due to the reduction in travel and a drop of US$40 billion in room revenue in 2020 (Bryant, 2020). Also, the pandemics negatively affected how tourists behaved and made decisions; rationally, they cancelled the trips that they had planned in fear of disease, since there is a high likelihood of catching viruses during travel (Park et al., 2019; Bauer et al., 2021). This is because tourists usually contribute significantly to transferring the existing or new variants of the virus to their destinations.

Various economies have relied on tourism as a poverty alleviation and economic growth promotion strategy, mostly in sub-Saharan Africa. The enhancement of the tourism sector has decreased the income disparity between wealthy and poorer countries/economies; the real per capita GDP growth averaged 2.4% from 1990 to 2019 for tourism-led economies like Seychelles and Mauritius, which is higher than in economies within sub-Saharan Africa that are not as much driven by tourism. However, Güvenek and Alptekin (2015) stated that tourists' motivation to visit a particular place is influenced by various factors, including the economic, political, and social stability of that country and above all, the natural and physical conditions of their destination. COVID-19 has created a negative impression about many destinations in terms of safety. It has led to the stagnation of arrivals, and this has brought about new dynamics in employment opportunities in some countries; the Seychelles has even tried to implement some plans to pay out-of-work tourism sector workers. This has led to declining revenues and even non-maintenance of specific tourist attractions. For example, the poor management of zoological tourist sites has left endangered species vulnerable to extinction.

Another consequence of the pandemic is the revenue losses realised from the tourism industry, which may push governments to re-strategise their public finance policy for the year. Usually, this translates to under-funding other budget items, especially those with immediate benefits such as environmentally related policies. In addition, some tourist destinations have ecotourism initiatives that encourage ecologically friendly activities, such as game reserves, national gardens/parks, and conservation zones, which are all good for the environment but have been disrupted by the pandemic. Moreover, there is physical damage to the environment, as evidence shows that The Caribbean Hotel and Tourism Association has projected that around 60% of the 30,000 new hotel rooms under construction within the Caribbean region will no longer be completed. These rooms were mainly targeted at accommodating tourists (Behsudi, 2020). Therefore, it is evident that pandemics usually disrupt tourist areas based on the environment and have a negative effect on it.

3.6 OPPORTUNITY COST OF THE FIGHT AGAINST CLIMATE CHANGE

The global resolve to fight climate change dates from a conference from 12 to 23 February 1979, in Geneva, sponsored by the World Meteorological Organization. It attracted scientists from all over the world to make up one of the leading international conferences on climate change, which led to the conception of the Intergovernmental Panel on Climate Change (IPCC) in 1988. Since then, several global responses to climate change have emerged, some of which include: the IPCC First Assessment Report of 1990, the Second World Climate Conference of 1990, approval of the start of treaty negotiations in December 1990 by the UN General Assembly, and the signing of the 1992 UN Framework Convention on Climate Change by 154 states in March 1994.

These all culminated in the birth of the annual international conference known as the Conference of the Parties (COP) in Berlin from 28 March to 7 April 1995. This first COP (COP 1) hosted over 2,000 delegates, observers, and journalists. Worthy of mention is the COP 15 Copenhagen Accord of 2009, where developed countries committed to jointly mobilise US$100 billion a year by 2020, which was formalised and reaffirmed in COP 16 in the Cancún, Mexico climate change conference of 2010. At COP 17 in Durban, South Africa, the Parties committed to mobilising US$100 billion annually by 2020, extending to 2025 in COP 21 in Paris (Huang and Guilanpour, 2021). These agreements and many more stem from the rapidly changing climate across the globe and its tremendous negative implications for us all.

The urgency and need to fund climate change adaptation and mitigation cannot be overemphasised. The global average surface temperature has changed drastically since the late 1930s, as shown below. The average surface temperature across land and ocean in 2020 was 1.02 °C, which is about ten times hotter than in 1938 (0 °C) and about 15 times hotter than in 1909, which recorded around −0.48 °C. The last 5 years have been the hottest in over 140 years. NASA's Gravity Recovery and Climate Experiment estimated that about 279 billion and 148 billion tons of ice were lost annually between 1993 and 2019 in Greenland and Antarctica, respectively (Velicogna et al., 2020). Furthermore, recent statistics on rising sea levels, ocean acidity, and wind speed enforce the argument for urgent action on climate change adaptation and mitigation (Figure 3.1).

Nevertheless, actual climate funding over the years shows that the 2009 Copenhagen accord has not been attained. The Climate Policy Initiative estimates that the total climate-related financing was about US$510 to US$530 billion in 2017 as against the expected US$800 billion (100 billion pledged for 8 years), while the UN's Framework Convention on Climate Change estimates it at US$681 billion in 2016 (Yeo, 2019). A United Nations 2019 report cited the UN Secretary-General António Guterres as concluding that 'the only realistic scenarios' showed the $100-billion target was out of reach and 'We are not there yet' (Bhattacharya et al., 2020). Furthermore, COP 26 recognised that climate funding contributions had failed to meet the 2020 target of $100 billion a year. This is not very encouraging, especially considering that the IPCC (2018) report posits that an estimated US$2.4 trillion is required annually for the energy sector alone by 2035 to curtail global warming below 1.5 ° in order to avert calamitous consequences.

Pandemics have a history of accelerating both private and public debts, leading to a surge in global debt. In 2020, total global debt increased from about 30% to 263% of GDP, the most significant single-year surge since 1970 (Kose et al., 2021). As the debt level increases, the interest rates on such debts also increase,

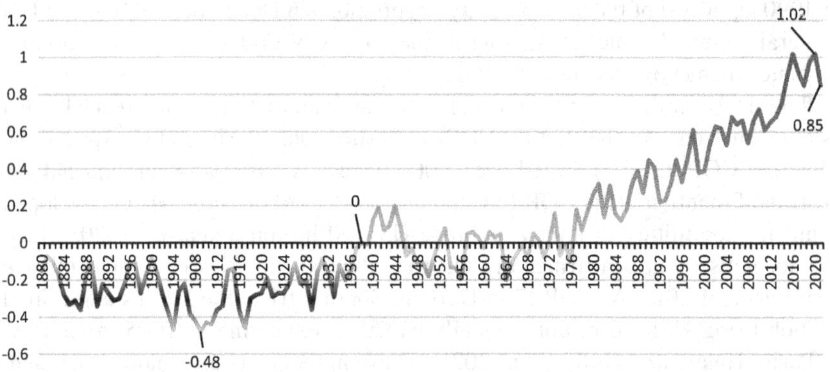

FIGURE 3.1 Global land-ocean temperature index. (From NASA Global Climate Change Signs of the Planet, 2022, https://climate.nasa.gov/vital-signs/global-temperature/.)

making debt servicing expensive; it is sometimes financed through higher taxes, increased borrowing, and reduced government expenditure. Reduction in government expenditure may extend to the reduction of essential activities such as social safety nets or growth-inducing public investment (Debrun and Kinda, 2016; Obstfeld, 2013; Reinhart and Rogoff, 2010). This is undoubtedly the case with sacrificing climate change funding at the end of the COVID-19 pandemic.

Given the economic implications of the COVID-19 pandemic, it is therefore expected that the inability to attain the agreed financial commitments may just have got worse. The fall in official development assistance (ODA) due to COVID-19 directly affects climate financing in developing countries. For example, the 0.7% gross national income (GNI) donor target for ODA set by the UN is legally binding in the UK but may drop due to the 11.5% decline forecast in GNI, while France was poised to set a target ODA of 0.55% of GNI but had to postpone due to COVID-19 (Donor Tracker, 2020; Quevedo et al., 2020). It is also expected that in some developed countries, the decline in climate aid may be much greater than the decline in GNI, especially where there is no budget restriction. Very conspicuous was the submission of the president of Seychelles, Wavel John Charles Ramkalawan, who lamented that COVID-19 had wiped away 75% of the proceeds of his country's tourism industry and therefore called for the adoption of a 'vulnerability index' over the income status criterion (International Institute for Sustainable Development, 2021). Consequently, the financial implications of COVID-19 will further cripple climate financing and therefore, the environment, at least in the short run.

In 2020, the United Nations Development Programme (UNDP) undertook a global study on public opinion about whether climate change is an emergent shock that must take priority. The findings suggested that two-thirds (67%) of the sample recognised it as a global emergency; hence, it has been given a closer eye, with the World Bank Group being the main funding body in this regard and having spent around $83 billion over the last 5 years. This breeds hope that individuals still perceive the reality of climate change and will still prioritise it. However, government institutions may also deal with the reality of scarce resources competing for serious budget items.

3.7 CONCLUSION

This chapter examines the economic outcomes of emerging pandemics, focusing on the COVID-19 pandemic, which is the most recent and has had arguably the most widespread impact. This chapter examines the effect on economic growth and financial flows, GVCs, global debts, ICT development, tourism and travel, and the opportunity cost of the fight against climate change. The study concludes that:

- Emerging pandemics such as SARS and COVID-19 had movement restrictions that affected economic wellbeing in East Asia in the case of SARS, with more severe consequences for economic growth and financial flows in the case of the COVID-19 pandemic. The considerable decline in economic growth after the COVID-19 outbreak is not unrelated to the degree of food wastage, which has dire effects on the environment

- The pandemic restrictions disrupted international trade, negatively affecting GVCs and the business sector. Furthermore, the disruption of GVCs due to pandemics tends to stimulate countries to be self-sufficient. This may create and maintain many more production plants that threaten the environment. In addition, previous heavy-weight production plants that were part of the GVCs incur huge wastes that emit carbon emissions into the atmosphere, increasing the pressure of global warming and climate change
- The movement restrictions and calls for self-isolation or quarantine had drastic effects on the tourism and travel industry. As a result, there was an evident decline in the revenues earned from this important sector, along with the high unemployment rate of workers from the tourism sector, and the governments had to give out relief packages to such households, money that could otherwise have been used in dealing with issues around climate change
- The COVID-19 pandemic significantly increased ICT usage thanks to the movement restrictions and closure of work and businesses. This could be recorded as a benefit of the pandemic, as increased use will improve efficiency in transactions, communications, and the development of financial inclusion, among others. The pandemic, however, reduced climate funding, and the increase in usage translates to more climate risks in the long run in terms of the production and powering of electronic appliances
- The 2009 Copenhagen accord succeeded in getting industrialised countries to pledge $US100 billion yearly for climate change adaptation and mitigation advancement in developing countries. So far, this pledge has not been met, as was acknowledged in COP 26. The COVID-19 pandemic further worsened the likelihood of this funding, as these industrialised nations had to respond to the immediate emergency at the expense of climate change adaptation and mitigation

Therefore, it is imperative to note that the economic outcomes of emerging pandemics – notably COVID-19 – have several environmental implications. There is a need to integrate institutional adaptation and mitigation strategies for pandemics with adaptation and mitigation strategies for the environment, regardless of the prevailing economic circumstances.

REFERENCES

Abbas, J., Mubeen, R., Terhemba-Iorember, P., Raza, S., and Mamirkulova, G. 2021. Exploring the impact of Covid-19 on tourism: Transformational potential and implications for a sustainable recovery of the travel and leisure industry. *Current Research in Behavioral Sciences,* 2, 100033. https://doi.org/10.1016/j.crbeha.2021.100033

Bauer, A., Garman, E., McDaid, D., Avendano, M., Hessel, P., Díaz,Y., Araya, R., Crick, C., Malvasi, P., Matijasevich, A., Park, A., Paula, C., Ziebold, C., Zimmerman, A., and Evans-Lacko, S. 2021. Integrating youth mental health into cash transfer programmes in response to the COVID-19 crisis in low-income and middle-income countries. *Lancet Psychiatry*. doi: 10.1016/S2215-0366(20)30382-5.

Behsudi, A. 2020. Tourism-dependent economies are among those harmed the most by the pandemic. *Finance & Development*.

Bhattacharya, A., Calland, R., Averchenkova, A., Gonzalez, L., Martinez-Diaz, L., and Van Rooij, J. 2020. Delivering on the $100 billion climate finance commitment and transforming climate finance. *Independent Group on Climate Financing*, December 2020. Available at https://www.un.org/sites/un2.un.org/files/100_billion_climate_finance_report.pdf.

Bonadio, B., Huo, Z., Levchenko, A., and Pandalai-Nayar, N. 2020. The role of global supply chains in the COVID-19 pandemic and beyond. *VoxEU.Org* (blog). May 25, 2020. https://voxeu.org/article/role-global-supply-chains-Covid-19-pandemic-and-beyond.

Branscombe, M. 2020. The network impact of the global COVID-19 pandemic. *The New Stack*. https://thenewstack.io/the-network-impact-of-the-global-Covid-19-pandemic/.

Bryant, B. 2020. The impact of COVID-19 on tourism. https://cnr.ncsu.edu/news/2020/07/impact-of-covid-19-on-tourism/.

De, R., Pandey, N., and Pal, A. 2020. Impact of digital surge during Covid-19 pandemic: A viewpoint on research and practice. *International Journal of Information Management*, 55, 102171. doi: 10.1016/j.ijinfomgt.2020.102171.

Debrun, X., and Kinda, T. 2016. That squeezing feeling: The interest burden and public debt stabilization. *International Finance*, 19(2), 147–178.

Donor Tracker. 2020. Independent analysis of 14 major OECD donors' official development assistance (ODA)- countries of focus in this report: United Kingdom, France, Germany, Netherlands, United States of America, and the European Commission. Berlin: SEEK Development.

Evenett, J. 2020. Chinese whispers: COVID-19, global supply chains in essential goods, and public policy. *Journal of International Business Policy*, 3, 408–429.

Filho, W. L., Voronova, V., Kloga, M., Paco Arminda, M. A., Salvia, A. L., Ferreira, C. D., and Subarna, S. 2021. COVID-19 and waste production in households: A trend analysis. *Science of the Total Environment*, 10(777). doi: 10.1016/j.scitotenv.2021.145997.

Fortune Business Insights. 2020. Impact of Covid-19 on information, communication and technology (ICT) market size, share, industry analysis and regional forecasts. https://www.fortunebusinessinsights.com/impact-of-Covid-19-on-information-communication-and-technology-ict-industry-102769.

Güvenek, B., and Alptekin, V. 2015. Turistlere yönelik terör saldırılarının turizme etkisi türkiye üzerine ampirik bir çalışma. *Selçuk Üniversitesi Sosyal Bilimler Meslek Yüksek Okulu Dergisi*, 17(1), 21–38.

Huang, J., and Guilanpour, K. 2021. Climate finance: Issues for COP 26. *Center for Climate and Energy Solutions*. chrome-extension://efaidnbmnnnibpcajpcglclefindmkaj/viewer.html?pdfurl=https%3A%2F%2Fwww.c2es.org%2Fwp-content%2Fuploads%2F2021%2F06%2FClimate-Finance-Issues-for-COP26.pdf&clen=216992&chunk=true.

ICTFOOTPRINT-EU. 2020. The impact of COVID is accelerating digital connectivity trend and it will influence the growth of the Information technology market in the near future. European framework initiative for energy & environmental efficiency in the ICT sector. https://ictfootprint.eu/en/news/environmental-impact-ict-reducing

-ict-footprint-and-rethinking-progress-technology#:~:text=All%20that%20glitters%20is%20not%20gold%20and%20switching,it%20uses%20and%20the%20cooling%20systems%20it%20requires.

International Institute for Sustainable Development. 2021, November 16. Glasgow climate change conference: October 31st – November 13th 2021. *Earth Negotiations Bulletin A Reporting Service for Environment and Development Negotiations*, 12(793), 1–40. https://enb.iisd.org/glasgow-climate-change-conference-cop26/summary-report.

IPCC. 2018. Global warming of 1.5°C. October 8, 2018. http://www.ipcc.ch/report/sr15/.

Kose, M. A., Nagle, P., Ohnsorge, F., and Sugawara, N. 2021. Debt tsunami of the pandemic. https://www.brookings.edu/blog/future-development/2021/12/17/debt-tsunami-of-the-pandemic/.

Matthes, J. 2020. Protektionismus Eindämmen und WTO-Reform Vorantreiben – Handelspolitische Empfehlungen für Bundesregierung und EU, Gutachten für die Initiative Neue Soziale Marktwirtschaft, Cologne.

NASA Global Climate Change Signs of the Planet. 2022. *Global Temperature*. Retrieved from https://climate.nasa.gov/vital-signs/global-temperature/.

Nay, I., and Shields, S. 2019. The 2003 severe acute respiratory syndrome epidemic: A retroactive examination of economic costs. Asian Development Bank Economics Working Paper Series, No 591.

Oberoi, P., and Singh, N. 2020. COVID-19: Consequences and opportunities for the ICT sector. https://fractal.ai/Covid-19-consequences-opportunities-for-ict/.

Obstfeld, M. 2013. On keeping your powder dry: Fiscal foundations of financial and price stability. *Monetary and Economic Studies*, 31, 25–37.

OECD. 2020. COVID-19 and global value chains: Policy options to build more resilient production networks. https://www.oecd.org/coronavirus/policy-responses/covid-19-and-global-value-chains-policy-options-to-build-more-resilient-production-networks-04934ef4/.

OECD. 2021. Global value chains: Efficiency and risks in the context of COVID-19. https://www.oecd.org/coronavirus/policy-responses/global-value-chains-efficiency-and-risks-in-the-context-of-covid-19-67c75fdc/.

Park, S., Boatwright, B., and Avery, E. J. 2019. Information channel preference in health crisis: Exploring the roles of perceived risk, preparedness, knowledge, and intent to follow directives. *Public Relations Review*, 45(5), 101794.

Quevedo, A., Peters, K., and Cao, Y. 2020. The impact of Covid-19 on climate change and disaster resilience funding. chrome-extension://efaidnbmnnnibpcajpcglclefindmkaj/viewer.html?pdfurl=https%3A%2F%2Fcdn.odi.org%2Fmedia%2Fdocuments%2FThe_impact_of_Covid-19_on_climate_change_and_disaster_resilience_funding_trends.pdf&clen=167934&chunk=true.

Reinhart, C. M., and Rogoff, K. S. 2010. Growth in a time of debt. *American Economic Review*, 100(2), 573–578.

Roberts, J. 2003. SARS outbreak deepens economic decline in South East Asia. June 2, 2003. https://www.wsws.org/en/articles/2003/06/sars-j02.html.

Seric, A., Görg, H., Mösle, S., and Windisch, M. 2020. How the pandemic disrupts global value chains: COVID-19 struck at the core of GVC hub regions, with severe implications for international production networks. https://iap.unido.org/articles/how-pandemic-disrupts-global-value-chains.

Sturgeon, J., and Memedović, O. 2011. Mapping global value chains: Intermediate goods trade and structural change in the world economy. United Nations Industrial Development Organization (UNIDO). Development Policy and Strategic Research Branch Working Paper 05/2010. https://www.unido.org/api/opentext/documents/download/9928658/unido-file-9928658.

The environmental impact of ICT: Reducing the ICT footprint and rethinking progress & technology with sustainability in mind. https://www.fortunebusinessinsights.com/impact-of-Covid-19-on-information-communication-and-technology-ict-industry-102769.

The Guardian News. 2020, April 9. 'A disastrous situation': Mountains of food wasted as coronavirus scrambles supply chain. https://www.theguardian.com/world/2020/apr/09/us-coronavirus-outbreak-agriculture-food-supply-waste.

The Wall Street Journal. 2020. Closed because of the Coronavirus, restaurants clear out their pantries. April 4, 2020. https://www.wsj.com/articles/closed-due-to-coronavirus-restaurants-clear-out-their-pantries-11586005203?mod=article_inline.

Tripp, S., and T. Partners. 2020. Response and resilience: Lessons learned from global life sciences ecosystems in the COVID-19 pandemic. Pittsburgh, Pennsylvania.

Twigby. 2020, May 28. U. S. study finds COVID-19 pandemic transforms cell phone usage. https://www.prnewswire.com/news-releases/us-study-finds-Covid-19-pandemic-transforms-cell-phone-usage-301066502.html.

United Nation World Trade Organisation. 2020. Tourism and Covid-19 – Unprecedented economic impacts. https://www.unwto.org/tourism-and-covid-19-unprecedented-economic-impacts.

United Nations Conference on Trade and Development. 2020. How COVID-19 is changing global value chains. https://unctad.org/news/how-covid-19-changing-global-value-chains.

United Nations Development Programme. 2020. COVID-19 and human development: Assessing the crisis, envisioning the recovery. 2020 Human Development Perspectives.

Velicogna, I., Mohajerani, Y., Geruo, A., Landerer, F., Mouginot, J., Noel, B., Rignot, E., Sutterly, T., van den Broeke, M., van Wessem, M., and Wiese, D. 2020. Continuity of Ice Sheet Mass Loss in Greenland and Antarctica from the GRACE and GRACE follow-on missions. *Geophysical Research Letters*, 47(8), e2020GL087291.

World Bank Indicators. 2022. Economy and growth. https://data.worldbank.org/topic/economy-and-growth?view=chart.

World Economic Forum. 2020. Here's how COVID-19 creates food waste mountains that threaten the environment. https://www.weforum.org/agenda/2020/06/Covid-19-food-waste-mountains-environment/.

Yeo, S. 2019. Where climate cash is flowing and why it's not enough. *Nature*. https://www.nature.com/articles/d41586-019-02712-3.

4 Tuberculosis
An Old Enemy of Mankind and Possible Next Pandemic

Chitra Rani, Raj Kishor Pandey, and Shah Ubaid-ullah

CONTENTS

4.1 Introduction 47
4.2 *Mycobacterium tuberculosis*: A Bug Responsible for TB 49
4.2.1 Transmission of TB and Its Progression Inside the Host 50
4.2.2 Therapeutics for TB 51
4.3 Air Pollution: an Alarming Situation for TB 53
4.3.1 Air Pollution: A Man-Made Disaster 53
4.3.2 Types of Pollutants 54
4.3.2.1 Particulate Matter 54
4.3.2.2 Carbon Monoxide (CO) 55
4.3.2.3 Nitrogen Dioxide (NO_2) 55
4.3.2.4 Ozone 55
4.3.2.5 Sulfur dioxide (SO_2) 56
4.3.2.6 Other Air Pollutants 56
4.4 The Role of Air Pollutants in TB Infection 57
4.5 Conclusion 58
References 58

4.1 INTRODUCTION

Tuberculosis (TB) is a malady that has haunted humanity for centuries and still continues to be a life-threatening disease. Globally, TB is a leading infectious disease, responsible for millions of deaths every year. The World Health Organization (WHO) in the year 1993 declared TB a global public health emergency; since then, it has been a major health concern for developing as well as developed countries (WHO, 1993). According to a WHO report, there were 10 million (range, 8.9–11.0 million) cases of TB and 1.2 million (range, 1.1–1.3 million) TB deaths in 2019 (WHO, 2020). Although a well-established

DOI: 10.1201/9781003288732-4

chemotherapy regimen is available for treatment, before the emergence of SARS-CoV-2, TB was the leading cause of mortality among infectious diseases. The most recent report on global TB cases, published by WHO in 2021, gives the details of TB cases for 2020, during the COVID-19 pandemic. According to this report, the number of deaths due to TB has increased for the first time in 9 years, and at the same time, there is a decline of 18% in the notification of TB cases as compared with previous years. This is due to the COVID-19 pandemic halting the services given to TB patients. According to the WHO, the geographical distribution of TB cases is as follows: South-East Asia (43%), Africa (25%), and the Western Pacific (18%), with smaller shares in the Eastern Mediterranean (8.3%), the Americas (3.0%), and Europe (2.3%). Thirty high-TB-burden countries account for 86% of all estimated incident cases worldwide, and eight of these countries (Figure 4.1) account for two-thirds of the global total: India (26%), China (8.5%), Indonesia (8.4%), the Philippines (6.0%), Pakistan (5.8%), Nigeria (4.6%), Bangladesh (3.6%), and South Africa (3.3%) (WHO, 2021).

TB is considered an old enemy of the human race, with the modern version being more dangerous and invincible. The primary or first line of treatment for the infection is a multidrug cocktail composed of rifampin (RIF), isoniazid (INH), pyrazinamide (PZA), and ethambutol (ETH). This regimen is recommended for at least 6 months to achieve high cure rates (WHO, 2010). With this course, TB has been cured successfully, but the use of multiple drugs

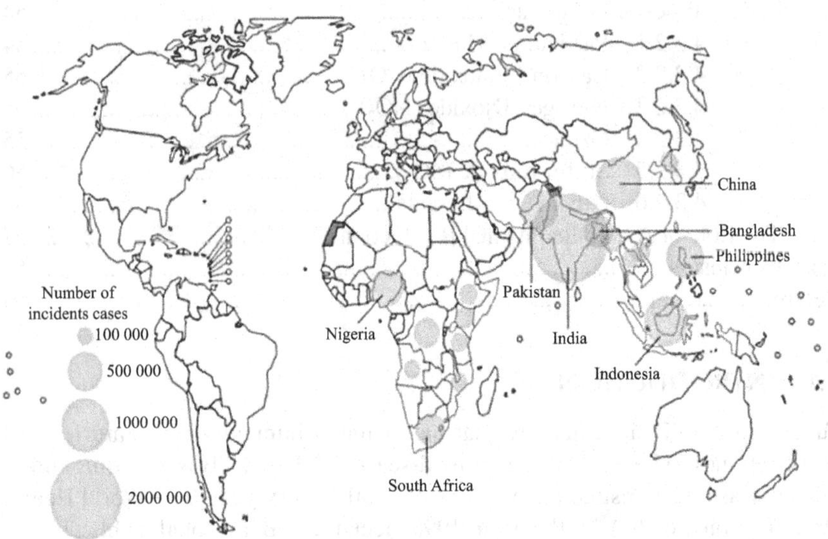

FIGURE 4.1 TB cases in 2020 for countries reporting at least 100,000 incident cases. Among all the countries, eight were highlighted that accounted for two-thirds of global TB cases. (From WHO, *Global Tuberculosis Report 2021*, World Health Organization, Geneva, 2021.)

risks non-compliance with the treatment, which ultimately leads to the development of drug-resistant-strains (DR). It was reported in 2019 that among half a million people who developed rifampicin-resistant TB (RR-TB), 78% had multidrug-resistant TB (MDR-TB) (WHO, 1993). These figures themselves explain the havoc caused by DR-TB worldwide. TB caused by *Mycobacterium tuberculosis*, a partial Gram-positive bacillus, mainly attacks the lungs, known as pulmonary TB, but the pathogen has the capability of infecting other sites, referred to as extra-pulmonary TB. A proper understanding of the associated risk factors is essential to plan strategies for controlling TB disease (Figure 4.1).

Different factors such as diabetes, alcohol, malnutrition, tobacco smoke, and air quality, which affect a large number of people, lead to acceleration in the progression of *M. tuberculosis* infection to full-blown TB (Narasimhan et al., 2013). Primarily, individual habitual activities are responsible for the progression of the disease, but human activities have had a negative impact on the environment in the recent years, like the degraded quality of the water we use, the quality of air we breathe, and the soil where vegetation is grown. As well as technological development, betterment of society, and providing valuable services to mankind, the industrial revolution resulted in large-scale production of pollutants in air and water, which are directly or indirectly hazardous to health. Air pollution because of anthropogenic activities is a serious health risk, responsible for around nine million deaths each year (WHO Air Pollution, 2021). There can be no doubt that these activities have a great impact on climate, and the repercussions of these factors in the event of some threat can be detrimental (Moore, 2009). Food safety challenges and food crises, melting of ice and icebergs, shrinking glaciers, and loss of flora and fauna are all severe results of climate change and the effects of global warming on diverse ecosystems (Karl et al., 2009; Marlon et al., 2019). In this chapter, the impact of air pollution on the progression of TB cases worldwide will be discussed.

4.2 *MYCOBACTERIUM TUBERCULOSIS*: A BUG RESPONSIBLE FOR TB

Among the 20 different mycobacterial species known to cause TB in humans, *M. tuberculosis* is the primary human pathogen. This bacterium is an obligate intracellular organism belonging to the *M. tuberculosis* complex (MTBC). The MBTC includes at least seven species of the genus Mycobacterium belonging to the family Mycobacteriaceae and order Actinomycetales (Ducati et al., 2006). In West Africa, about 50% of TB infection is caused by *M. africanum*. A less common form of human TB is caused by *M. canetti* in Eastern Africa. In cattle, TB is caused by *M. bovis* and *M. caprae* species (Bos et al., 2014). The transmission of TB from animals to humans occurs through direct contact with animals or consuming unpasteurised milk. It has been reported that other Mycobacterium species may be responsible for zoonotic TB in humans, for example *M. microti*, a pathogen for rodents (Kispar et al., 2014), and *M. pinnipedii*, a pathogen for seals (Cousins et al., 2003). Among all the species of Mycobacterium, only *M. tuberculosis* and *M. africanum* are predominately responsible for TB in humans.

M. tuberculosis, an aerobic, non-spore-forming, motile bacterium, possesses a cell wall having a high proportion of high-molecular-weight lipids. It is a slow-growing microbe, having a doubling time of 15–20 hours, while for most common bacterial pathogens, it is less than 1 hour. In solid media, visible growth takes 3–8 weeks. This microbe tends to grow in parallel groups, creating characteristic colonies of serpentine strings. As compared with other bacteria, in *M. tuberculosis* a good percentage of genes encode for proteins involved in lipogenesis and lipolysis (Delogu et al., 2013; Smith, 2003).

4.2.1 Transmission of TB and Its Progression Inside the Host

M. tuberculosis follows an established route of contagion. When a few tubercle bacilli, spread in air from an infected person having active pulmonary TB, reach the alveoli of the host by inhalation of contaminated air, this leads to primary *M. tuberculosis* infection. The entry of *M. tuberculosis* is mediated by several receptors presented on the surface of host cells, such as Toll-like receptors, nucleotide-binding oligomerisation domain-2 (NOD-2) like receptors (NLRs), and C-type lectins (Danelishvili et al., 2003; García-Pérez et al., 2003). Upon encountering the pathogen attack, the host presents a complex series of layered defences. This multi-layered defence mechanism includes non-specific mucosal barriers and non-antigenic-specific phagocytosis, leading ultimately to specific immune responses by antigen-presenting cells, which include dendritic cells (DCs), macrophages, and B lymphocytes orchestrated by antigen-specific T and B lymphocytes through cytokine signalling, cytotoxic T cell function, and antibody production. *M. tuberculosis* is quickly phagocytosed by the alveolar macrophages, initiating the innate immune response, which has potential to destroy the invading bacteria (Urdahl et al., 2011; Russell et al., 2001; Chan et al., 2004). When *M. tuberculosis* enters host macrophages, initially it lives inside the endocytic vacuoles known as the phagosomes. In the next step, the phagosomal maturation cycle starts, where phagosome–lysosome fusion occurs. Here, *M. tuberculosis* encounters adverse conditions such as acidic pH, reactive oxygen intermediates, lysosomal enzymes, and toxic peptides. The reactive nitrogen intermediates (RNIs) mainly show antimicrobial activity against engulfed *M. tuberculosis* inside the alveolar macrophages (Nathan et al., 1991). It has been established that mice having mutations in the genes encoding the macrophage-localised cytokine inducible nitric oxide synthase are more vulnerable to various intracellular pathogens, including *Leishmania major* (Wei et al., 1995), *Listeria monocytogenes* (MacMicking et al., 1995), and *M. tuberculosis* (MacMicking et al., 1997). In the case of *M. tuberculosis* infection, it has been recognised that in mouse macrophages, RNIs are the most important weapon against virulent mycobacteria. It was observed that resistance to RNIs among different strains of *M. tuberculosis* is directly linked with the severity of the infection (Chan et al., 1995; Chan et al., 1992; O'Brien et al., 1994). Although the role of RNIs as antimicrobial agents against *M. tuberculosis* in the mouse model is defined clearly, the same mechanism in human macrophages and its potential role are debatable (Nicholson et al., 1996). The majority of TB cases among the human population showed inducible nitric oxide synthase activity inside alveolar macrophages. Although the host defence mechanism has the capability to get rid of the bacterial infection at the early stage, *M. tuberculosis* has developed a mechanism to escape engulfment by the macrophages, and it starts actively replicating in peculiar structures called granulomas, formed by macrophages along with epithelioid cells and multinucleated cells known as Langhans' giant cells and T lymphocytes (Flynn et al., 2001; Flynn et al., 2003). The population of *M. tuberculosis* survives the host's immune response and persists in a non-replicating state called latent TB infection (Tufariello et al., 2003). Pro-inflammatory and anti-inflammatory cytokine production has to be blocked for establishment of TB infection. For increased shielding function of the granuloma, tumour necrosis factor α (TNF-α), interferon-γ (IFN-γ), and interleukin (IL)-1β have an important role, whereas IL-10 is a negative regulator for inflammatory response (Kaisho et al., 2000; Aderem et al., 2000). The function of TNF-α is to enhance granuloma formation, while IFN-γ boosts antigen presentation and employment of CD4+ T cells or CD8+ cells, thus mediating the killing of bacteria. The secretion of these cytokines is initiated by specific pathogen-associated molecular patterns (PAMS) recognised by pattern recognition receptors (PRRs) that are specific for some signature molecules belonging to *M. tuberculosis*. Upon detection of specific PAMS by PRRs that sense *M. tuberculosis* signature molecules, a variety of cytokines are secreted and regulated by macrophages and DCs. The PRRs are responsible for triggering both innate (non-specific) as well as adaptive (specific) immune response to *M. tuberculosis* (Akira et al., 2006).

4.2.2 Therapeutics for TB

In the olden days, sanatoria were established to manage and treat TB patients. In 1854, the first sanatoria were established in Western Europe and America. Sanatoria were very commonly found at that time throughout Europe and the US, and served dual functions. First, they provided protection to the general population by isolating the sick persons who were the source of infection. Second, they offered bed rest, exercise, fresh air, and good nutrition to individuals infected with *M. tuberculosis* (Palomino, 2007). Surgical procedures were also commonly used as treatment tools for TB patients, such as artificial pneumothorax, phrenicectomy, or thoracoplasty, in which clean and filtered air was introduced into the pleural spaces of the lungs (Sharpe, 1931). The invention of Bacille Calmette-Guérin (BCG) marked a historic event that brought optimism to fighting TB, particularly in endemic areas (Calmette et al., 1921). These strategies were used to tackle TB cases before the antibiotic era, but after the discovery of streptomycin in 1943 by A. Schatz and S. Waksman, the preliminary steps were taken toward the development of anti-TB drugs. Streptomycin was isolated from cultures of *Streptomyces griseus*. Streptomycin inhibited the growth of *M. tuberculosis* in laboratory animals with low toxicity (Jones et al., 1944; Schatz et al., 1944). For this discovery, S. Waksman won the 1952 Nobel Prize in the field of physiology or medicine. But, this phenomenal breakthrough came to an early end because of the emergence of streptomycin-resistant *M. tuberculosis* strains. After this, other anti-TB drugs, like *p*-aminosalicylic acid (Nagley et al., 1949), isoniazid (Robitzek et al., 1952), ethambutol (Thomas et al., 1961), rifampin (Sensi, 1983), pyrazinamide (McKenzie et al., 1948), and cycloserine (MH et al., 1955), were discovered. It was shown that the problem of drug resistance could be prevented by using a combination of two or three drugs. A standard regimen for the treatment of TB includes INH, RIF, ETH, and PZA for 2 months followed by INH and RIF for 4 months (WHO, 2010). Although multidrug therapy was successful for the treatment of TB patients infected with drug-sensitive *M. tuberculosis*, it was linked with other complications, such as longevity and toxicity; thus, the response was minimal, with the chance of failure and relapse, development of drug-resistant strains, and non-stop transmission of the infection. To address these concerns, the WHO recommended the DOTS (directly observed treatment, short-course) strategy to make sure that the patient follows the treatment without any failure so as to eradicate TB completely (Elzinga et al., 2004; Volmink et al., 2007). The DOTS programme is based on five basic fundamentals: political commitment, microscopic services, drug supplies, surveillance systems, and direct treatment observation. The programme has been effective in preventing the spread of new infection, as it helped to minimise the emergence of MDR-TB. Based on the mechanism of action and the associated side-effects, anti-TB drugs have been classified into two categories. The anti-TB drugs that represent the first-line treatment consist of INH, RIF, ETH, and PZA. The second line, which are both less effective and associated with side-effects, comprise fluoroquinolones (levofloxacin, moxifloxacin, gatifloxacin), three injectable drugs (amikacin, kanamycin, or capreomycin), ethionamide, and cycloserine (WHO, 2009). For MDR-TB, second-line drugs are used for up to 2 years. Non-compliance and the associated side-effects have resulted in the evolution of extensively drug-resistant TB (XDR-TB) (resistant to all four first-line drugs along with resistance to at least one second-line injectable and a fluoroquinolone) (Pasqualoto et al., 2001). Thus, a constant and continued effort is required for cure and management of MDR and XDR-TB. Therefore, a new regimen has been developed and implemented. In 2018, it was recommended that long-term treatment of MDR-TB should be done with oral therapeutics, and injectables should be avoided for an extended period (Murphy, 2018). This has been possible with the discovery of new anti-TB drugs, such as TMC207 and delamanid with the addition of linezolid, which was previously in use for the treatment of other diseases. A year later, in 2019, a new regimen was approved for the cure and management of XDR and MDR-TB. It is a 6-month oral therapy comprising TMC207, pretomanid, and linezolid (Silva et al., 2020).

4.3 AIR POLLUTION: AN ALARMING SITUATION FOR TB

With the advancement of technology and development, various health problems are arising due to lifestyle changes and the utilisation of our environment for fulfilment of our needs. Worldwide increasing air pollution is a major concern for every nation, as it has a direct impact on public health. Exposure to ambient and indoor air pollution enhances the risk of pulmonary TB (Yao et al., 2019). Therefore, in this section, this important factor and its associated consequences for the lungs (the primary site for TB infection) will be discussed in detail.

4.3.1 Air Pollution: A Man-Made Disaster

During the first WHO Global Conference on Air Pollution and Health in 2018, Dr Tedros Adhanom Ghebreyesus, the Director General of WHO, described air pollution as a 'silent public health emergency' and 'the new tobacco' (Gatari et al., 2019). Causes of air pollution include both natural as well as man-made sources. The latter have become a leading cause due to the industrial revolution. The significant contributors to air pollution are burning of fossil fuels and biomass for different purposes, such as powering means of transport and generating electricity; burning agricultural wastes or burning wastes in urban cities; and uncontrolled forest fires. Construction activities and re-suspension of surface dust are two more factors contributing to pollution. Further, air pollution is aggravated by atmospheric transport of contaminants from far-away sources. Air pollution is a most important health concern for everyone in developing or developed nations. According to one estimate, air pollution was responsible for 6.7 million premature deaths globally in 2019. This was because of exposure to fine particulate matter ($PM_{2.5}$) having a diameter of 2.5 μm or less, responsible for cardiovascular and respiratory diseases and different types of cancer. The impact of air pollution is greater in developing countries. The highest numbers have been seen in the South-East Asia and Western Pacific regions, implicated in 91% of the 4.2 million premature deaths reported (Fuller et al., 2022). Recent numbers also illustrate the direct effect of air pollution on cardiovascular diseases. In 2016, the WHO estimated that ischaemic heart disease and stroke accounted for 58% of premature deaths because of air pollution, whereas chronic obstructive pulmonary disease and acute lower respiratory infections accounted for 18% and lung cancer for 6%, respectively. For some deaths, more than one factor is involved. For lung cancer, both smoking and air pollution are contributory factors. Thus, in these cases, improving air quality or reducing or quitting smoking could prevent some deaths. Indoor smoke generated by cooking and heating using biomass like coal, wood, or dung as fuel is also a severe health problem for approximately 2.6 billion people. Indoor air pollution due to inefficient use of solid fuels or kerosene for cooking was responsible for 3.8 million premature deaths in 2016 (Figure 4.2) from low- and middle-income countries. Household air pollution is a major factor responsible for degrading air quality in both rural and urban locations and may

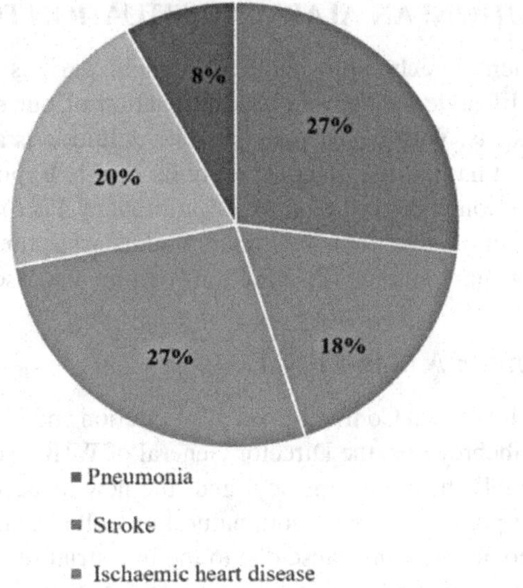

FIGURE 4.2 Percentage of deaths due to diseases caused by indoor pollution. (From World Health Organization, 2021 *WHO global air quality guidelines: Particulate matter (PM2.5 and PM10), ozone, nitrogen dioxide, sulfur dioxide and carbon monoxide*, ISBN: 978924003422,300).

account for up to 50% in some parts of world (WHO, 2016 and Ambient air pollution WHO, 2021).

4.3.2 Types of Pollutants

Several pollutants are mentioned by WHO as potential source of risk for human health, which are harmful for the environment and also cause damage to property. These include particulate matter (PM), carbon monoxide (CO), ozone (O_3), nitrogen dioxide (NO_2), and sulfur dioxide (SO_2). The severity of the disease depends upon the length of exposure to these various pollutants (Types of pollutants WHO, 2021).

4.3.2.1 Particulate Matter

PM is defined as particles that can be inhaled, made of sulfate, nitrates, ammonia, sodium chloride, black carbon, mineral dust, or water. It is an accepted substitute indicator of air pollution. Among all the different types of pollutants, it is the most harmful to human health. Depending on the aerodynamic diameter, PM is classified as PM_{10} (inhalable particles having a diameter less than 10 μm), $PM_{2.5}$ (fine particulate matter having a diameter less than 2.5

μm), and $PM_{0.1}$ (ultrafine particulate matter with a diameter less than 0.1 μm). The majority of PM pollution comes from man-made sources, including power plants, industry, domestic wood and coal burning, and cars. Natural sources include dust, sea salt, and wildfires. $PM_{2.5}$ is considered to be the most harmful of all particulate matter. This is because of its large surface area and its ability to adsorb different toxic and harmful substances. Due to the small size of $PM_{2.5}$, these particles reach the terminal bronchioles and alveoli and even have the potential to cross the gas–blood barrier to reach the circulatory system. Data collected from outpatient and emergency departments and hospitalisations because of respiratory infections shows a direct link between exposure to $PM_{2.5}$ and both upper and lower respiratory tract infections. Susceptibility to respiratory infections in children and the elderly increases because of exposure to $PM_{2.5}$. In a case-study involving lower respiratory tract infections due to $PM_{2.5}$, it was evident that 77% of these patients were infants aged between 0 and 2 years, and the main cause of infection was respiratory syncytial virus and influenza virus (Yang et al., 2020).

4.3.2.2 Carbon Monoxide (CO)

Partial combustion of fossil fuels results in the emission of CO into the atmosphere. CO is a colourless, odourless, and tasteless toxic gas that easily diffuses into the lung tissues and bloodstream, competing with oxygen for binding to the body's cells. It is already established that CO has a higher binding affinity for haemoglobin as compared with oxygen. As a result of this, the supply of oxygen to the lung tissues is affected, causing hypoxia, ischaemia, and cardiovascular diseases (Types of pollutants WHO, 2021).

4.3.2.3 Nitrogen Dioxide (NO_2)

NO_2 is considered as a highly reactive gas belonging to the nitrogen oxides (NOx) group. Nitrate aerosols are the prime source of NO_2, and it forms an essential fraction of $PM_{2.5}$. NO_2 is also an important precursor for ozone in the presence of ultraviolet light. Heating, power generation, and engines in vehicles and ships are the major sources of emissions of NO_2. The human respiratory system airways may become irritated when breathing air contaminated with NO_2. According to epidemiological research conducted by the WHO, prolonged NO_2 exposure is linked to an increase in bronchitis symptoms in children with asthma. NO_2 values now observed in cities in Europe and North America are likewise associated with reduced lung function and growth (Types of pollutants WHO, 2021; Hamra et al., 2015).

4.3.2.4 Ozone

Ozone, triplet oxygen (O_3), is created when a single oxygen atom (O), formed by splitting of oxygen (O_2) by absorbing energy from UV rays, reacts with dioxygen (O_2, the regular oxygen molecule). Ozone is present naturally in both the stratosphere and the troposphere. But, the higher levels of ozone are because of photochemical reactions involving volatile organic compounds and oxides of nitrogen (NOx: NO and NO_2). Ozone in air is also responsible for adverse respiratory effects, such as shortness of breath, pain when taking a deep breath, and inflammation of the air passages, in the general population. This may exacerbate asthma, emphysema, and chronic bronchitis (COPD). The respiratory health of children is at a high risk because of exposure to ozone, as children inhale a higher dose per unit of body mass, and their lungs have not developed completely. Ozone, a strong oxidising agent, leads to oxidative damage to cells, and it has been revealed that innate immunity is involved in ozone-induced inflammation of the respiratory tract, like the involvement of innate lymphoid cells in mice (Types of pollutants WHO, 2021; Zhang et al., 2019).

4.3.2.5 Sulfur dioxide (SO_2)

Sulfur dioxide is a colourless gas with a pungent odour. It is evolved from natural activities. Volcanic eruptions and combustion of biomass are the two major biogenic sources of SO_2 production. Oxidation of reduced sulfur species from biodegradation of organic material rich in sulfur compounds also produces SO_2, as does anaerobic reduction of sulfate (SO_4^{2-}). Combustion of fossil fuels, particularly coal and oil, electric items, and industry produce more than 90% of the SO_2 present in the atmosphere. It directly affects lung function and also causes eye irritation. It leads to inflammation of the respiratory tract, causing cough and mucus secretion, intensifying asthma and chronic bronchitis, and rendering people more susceptible to respiratory tract infections. Hospitalisations because of cardiac disease and associated mortality increase when SO_2 levels are high. On combining with H_2O, SO_2 forms H_2SO_4, which is the main cause of acid rain (Chen et al., 2007; Manisalidis et al., 2020).

4.3.2.6 Other Air Pollutants

Black carbon, polycyclic aromatic hydrocarbons (PAH), and methane are some other air pollutants that affect human health. Long-term exposure to PAH is linked with lung cancer. As we discussed, both outdoor air pollutants, which are mostly released due to combustion, air pollutants emitted indoors, and air pollution from non-combustion sources all have negative health impacts (Types of pollutants WHO, 2021). Radon is one example.

Radon is a radioactive gas, emitted by certain rock and soil formations, and it accumulates in the basement or ground levels of homes when there are insufficient ventilation or evacuation systems. Recently, it has been demonstrated that concentrated indoor radon is responsible for lung cancers in Europe, North America, and Asia. It accounts for 3% to 14% of cases, making radon a primary cause of lung cancer among non-smokers (Types of pollutants WHO, 2021; Somet et al., 2000).

The Air Quality Guidelines given by WHO (Global air quality guideline WHO, 2021) provide global recommendations on important air contaminants that pose health concerns, including thresholds and restrictions. The Guidelines are applicable to both outdoor and indoor environments worldwide and are based on expert evaluation of current scientific evidence (Table 4.1):

TABLE 4.1
Concentrations of various pollutants in the air for different averaging times (WHO, 2021)

Pollutant	Averaging time (mean)	Air quality guideline (μg/m³)
$PM_{2.5}$	Annual	10
$PM_{2.5}$	24-hour	25
PM_{10}	24-hour	20
PM_{10}	Annual	50
Ozone	8-hour	100
Nitrogen dioxide	Annual	40
Nitrogen dioxide	1-hour	200
Sulfur dioxide	24-hour	20
Sulfur dioxide	10-minute	500

4.4 THE ROLE OF AIR POLLUTANTS IN TB INFECTION

According to studies conducted in Los Angeles and northern California (US), exposure to a higher level of $PM_{2.5}$, CO, and NO_2 is linked with TB cases (Jassal et al., 2013; Smith et al., 2016). Air pollutants interfere with the immune response generated against the TB infection, which ultimately helps *M. tuberculosis* to replicate and survive inside the host cell. The diesel exhaust particles (DEP) released in the air due to industrial activities in urban areas are a major component of inhaled $PM_{2.5}$, which is deposited in the lungs. When a person is infected with TB, the macrophages present the first line of defence against the bacterium, but $PM_{2.5}$ deposited inside lung alveoli suppresses the macrophages' activity (Hiramatsu et al., 2005; Sarkar et al., 2012). Demarest and co-workers studied macrophages isolated within 36 hours of smoke inhalation in humans. They reported increased numbers of cells obtained by lavage from the lungs of smoke-exposed subjects (largely polymorphonuclear leukocytes) and decreased migration of pulmonary macrophages in response to a standard chemotactic stimulus (Demarest et al., 1979). Experimentally, it has been proven that DEP increases the pulmonary *M. tuberculosis* load because of low levels of production of pro-inflammatory cytokines (e.g., IL-1β, IL-12p40, and IFN-γ). The increased level of SO_2 also interferes with pulmonary defences such as alveolar macrophage function, mucociliary transport, and alveolar clearance. When 12.5 ppm of SO_2 exposure was given under *in vitro* conditions, it resulted in the death of 62% of alveolar macrophages, and there was a 63% reduction in reactive oxygen species. Exposure to SO_2 decreases the production of TNF-α and IL-1. Like SO_2, NO_2 also exploits the host body's immune response developed against TB. It has been reported that NO_2 inhibits the production of serum neutralising antibodies and phagocytosis of alveolar macrophages and blood mononuclear cells. Air pollution is responsible for not only drug-sensitive TB cases but also an increased incidence of DR-TB.

According to published experimental results, exposure to $PM_{2.5}$ for 540 days had a detrimental effect, and it was highly associated with an increase in cases of DR-TB. The same study also demonstrated the effects of other air pollutants on DR-TB (Sarkar et al., 2012; Yang et al., 2020; Yao et al., 2019).

There are various immunological indicators of TB infection, such as granulocyte macrophage-colony stimulating factor (GM-CSF), TNF-α, IFN, IL, and $CD4^+$ T cells. Among these, TNF-α, IFN, IL, and $CD4^+$ T cells are affected by air pollution (Yang et al., 2020). This correlation between air pollutants and the body's immune system, especially TB infection, needs to be investigated further.

4.5 CONCLUSION

The numbers of individuals infected with TB are increasing every year, and the emergence of DR-TB patients has raised concerns about the disease. The recent SARS-CoV-2 pandemic is an eye-opener for health authorities globally and also a warning that if already existing life-threatening diseases are not treated or controlled in time, these will emerge as another pandemic. Exposure of TB-infected people to polluted air is a serious health concern. Maintaining good air quality would aid the global TB control programme, and for complete eradication of TB, identifying different risk factors and how to control them is a primary step. Giving up smoking and the use of clean sources of energy will greatly facilitate decreasing indoor and outdoor air pollution and will prove helpful in controlling TB in developing countries to a great extent. To this end, international collaboration in the field of research, development, policy making, and monitoring is important for combating and reducing air pollution. An effective plan needs to be formulated by the collective approach of administration, different organisations, and healthcare professionals to control the situation. The public must be educated by professionals in the field and made aware of the different issues concerning pollution, particularly air pollution, so that the emergence of any problem is averted.

REFERENCES

Aderem, A., Ulevitch, R.J., 2000. Toll-like receptors in the induction of the innate immune response. *Nature* 406(6797), 782–787.

Akira, S., Uematsu, S., Takeuchi, O., 2006. Pathogen recognition and innate immunity. *Cell* 124(4), 783–801.

Ambient (Outdoor) Air Pollution. WHO. Available online at https://www.who.int/news-room/fact-sheets/detail/ambient-(outdoor)-air-quality-and-health (accessed on July 8, 2022).

Bos, K.I., Harkins, K.M., Herbig, A., Coscolla, M., Weber, N., Comas, I., Forrest, S.A., Bryant, J.M., Harris, S.R., Schuenemann, V.J., Campbell, T.J., Majander, K., Wilbur, A.K., Guichon, R.A., Wolfe Steadman, D.L., Cook, D.C., Niemann, S., Behr, M.A., Zumarraga, M., Bastida, R., Huson, D., Nieselt, K., Young, D., Parkhill, J., Buikstra, J.E., Gagneux, S., Stone, A.C., Krause, J., 2014. Pre-Columbian mycobacterial genomes reveal seals as a source of new world human tuberculosis. *Nature* 514(7523), 494–497.

Calmette, A., Boquet, A., Negre, L., 1921. Contribution à l'étude du bacille tuberculeux bilié. *Ann. Inst. Pasteur* 9, 561–570.

Chan, J., Flynn, J., 2004. The immunological aspects of latency in tuberculosis. *Clin. Immunol.* 110(1), 2–12.

Chan, J., Xing, Y., Magliozzo, R.S., Bloom, B.R., 1992. Killing of virulent Mycobacterium tuberculosis by reactive nitrogen intermediates produced by activated murine macrophages. *J. Exp. Med.* 175(4), 1111–1122.

Chan, J., Tanaka, K., Carroll, D., Flynn, J., Bloom, B.R., 1995. Effects of nitric oxide synthase inhibitors on murine infection with Mycobacterium tuberculosis. *Infect. Immun.* 63(2), 736–740.

Charles, E., Mckenna, M.H., Morton, R.F., 1955. Studies on the absorption, diffusion, and excretion of cycloserine. *Antibiot. Annu.* 3, 169–172.

Chen, T.M., Kuschner, W.G., Gokhale, J., Shofer, S., 2007. Outdoor air pollution: Nitrogen dioxide, sulfur dioxide, and carbon monoxide health effects. *Am. J. Med. Sci.* 333(4), 249–256.

Cousins, D.V., Bastida, R., Cataldi, A., Quse, V., Redrobe, S., Dow, S., Duignan, P., Murray, A., Dupont, C., Ahmed, N., Collins, D.M., Butler, W.R., Dawson, D., Rodríguez, D., Loureiro, J., Romano, M.I., Alito, A., Zumarraga, M., Bernardelli, A., 2003. Tuberculosis in seals caused by a novel member of the Mycobacterium tuberculosis complex: *Mycobacterium pinnipedii* sp. nov. *Int. J. Syst. Evol. Microbiol.* 53(5), 1305–1314.

Danelishvili, L., McGarvey, J., Li, Y.J., Bermudez, L.E., 2003. Mycobacterium tuberculosis infection causes different levels of apoptosis and necrosis in human macrophages and alveolar epithelial cells. *Cell. Microbiol.* 5(9), 649–660.

Delogu, G., Sali, M., Fadda, G., 2013. The biology of mycobacterium tuberculosis infection. *Mediterr. J. Hematol. Infect. Dis.* 5(1), e2013070. doi: 10.4084/MJHID.2013.070.

Demarest, G.B., Hudson, L.D., Altman, L.C., 1979. Impaired alveolar macrophage chemotaxis in patients with acute smoke inhalation. *Am. Rev. Respir. Dis.* 119(2), 279–286.

Ducati, R.G., Ruffino-Netto, A., Basso, L.A., Santos, D.S., 2006. The resumption of consumption: A review on tuberculosis. *Mem. Inst. Oswaldo Cruz* 101(7), 697–714.

Elzinga, G., Raviglione, M.C., Maher, D., 2004. Scale up: Meeting targets in global tuberculosis control. *Lancet* 363(9411), 814–819.

Flynn, J.L., Chan, J., 2001. Immunology of tuberculosis. *Annu. Rev. Immunol.* 19, 93.

Flynn, J.L., Chan, J., 2003. Immune evasion by Mycobacterium tuberculosis: Living with the enemy. *Curr. Opin. Immunol.* 15(4), 450–455.

Fuller, R., Landrigan, P.J., Balakrishnan, K., Bathan, G., Bose-O'Reilly, S., Brauer, M., Caravanos, J., Chiles, T., Cohen, A., Corra, L., Cropper, M., Ferraro, G., Hanna, J., Hanrahan, D., Hu, H., Hunter, D., Janata, G., Kupka, R., Lanphear, B., Lichtveld, M., Martin, K., Mustapha, A., Sanchez-Triana, E., Sandilya, K., Schaefli, L., Shaw, J., Seddon, J., Suk, W., Téllez-Rojo, M.M., Yan, C., 2022. Pollution and health: A progress update. *Lancet Planet Health* 6(6), e535–e547. doi: 10.1016/S2542-5196(22)00090-0. Erratum in: *Lancet Planet Health*, 2022 June 14; PMID: 35594895.

García-Pérez, B.E., Mondragón-Flores, R., Luna-Herrera, J., 2003. Internalization of Mycobacterium tuberculosis by macropinocytosis in non-phagocytic cells. *Microb. Pathog.* 35(2), 49–55.

Gatari, M.J., 2019. First WHO global conference on air pollution and health: A brief report. *Clean Air J.*, 29(1), 7.

Hamra, G.B., Laden, F., Cohen, A.J., Raaschou-Nielsen, O., Brauer, M., Loomis, D., 2015. Lung cancer and exposure to nitrogen dioxide and traffic: A systematic review and meta-analysis. *Environ. Health Perspect.* 123(11), 1107–1112.

Hiramatsu, K., Saito, Y., Sakakibara, K., Azuma, A., Kudoh, S., Takizawa, H., Sugawara, I., 2005. The effects of inhalation of diesel exhaust on murine mycobacterial infection. *Exp. Lung Res.* 31(4), 405–415. https://www.dreamstime.com/tuberculosis-life-cycle-mycobacterium-infection-caused-bacteria-infected-person-bacterium-able-to-reproduce-inside-image169684804.

Jassal, M.S., Bakman, I., Jones, B., 2013. Correlation of ambient pollution levels and heavily-trafficked roadway proximity on the prevalence of smear-positive tuberculosis. *Public Health* 127(3), 268–274.

Jones, D., Metzger, H.J., Schatz, A., Waksman, S.A., 1944. Control of gram-negative bacteria in experimental animals by streptomycin. *Science* 100(2588), 103–105.

Kaisho, T., Akira, S., 2000. Critical roles of toll-like receptors in host defense. *Crit. Rev. Immunol.* 20(5), 393–405.

Karl, T.R., Melillo, J.M., Peterson, T.C., Hassol, S.J. eds., 2009. *Global Climate Change Impacts in the United States.* Cambridge: Cambridge University Press.

Kipar, A., Burthe, S.J., Hetzel, U., Rokia, M.A., Telfer, S., Lambin, X., Birtles, R.J., Begon, M., Bennett, M., 2014. Mycobacterium microti tuberculosis in its maintenance host, the field vole (Microtus agrestis) characterization of the disease and possible routes of transmission. *Vet. Pathol.* 51(5), 903–914.

MacMicking, J.D., Nathan, C., Hom, G., Chartrain, N., Fletcher, D.S., Trumbauer, M., Stevens, K., Xie, Q.W., Sokol, K., Hutchinson, N., Chen, H., 1995. Altered responses to bacterial infection and endotoxic shock in mice lacking inducible nitric oxide synthase. *Cell* 81(4), 641–650.

MacMicking, J.D., North, R.J., LaCourse, R., Mudgett, J.S., Shah, S.K., Nathan, C.F., 1997. Identification of nitric oxide synthase as a protective locus against tuberculosis. *Proc. Natl. Acad. Sci. U. S. A.* 94(10), 5243–5248.

Manisalidis, I., Stavropoulou, E., Stavropoulos, A., Bezirtzoglou, E., 2020. Environmental and health impacts of air pollution: A review. *Front. Public Health.* 20(8), 14. doi: 10.3389/fpubh.2020.00014.

Marlon, J.R., Bloodhart, B., Ballew, M.T., Rolfe-Redding, J., Roser-Renouf, C., Leiserowitz, A., Maibach, E., 2019. How hope and doubt affect climate change mobilization. *Front. Commun.* 20. doi: 10.3389/fcomm.2019.00020.

McKenzie, D., Malone, L., Kushner, S., Oleson, J.J., Subbarow, Y., 1948. The effect of nicotinic acid amide on experimental tuberculosis of white mice. *J. Lab. Clin. Med.* 33(10), 1249–1253.

Moore, F.C., 2009. Climate change and air pollution: Exploring the synergies and potential for mitigation in industrializing countries. *Sustainability* 1(1), 43–54.

Murphy, D., 2018. Multidrug resistant TB: Fully oral regimens should help improve compliance, says WHO. *BMJ* 362, k3610. doi: 10.1136/bmj.

Nagley, M.M., Logg, M.H., 1949. Para-aminosalicylic acid (PAS) in pulmonary tuberculosis. *Lancet*, 253, 913–916.

Narasimhan, P., Wood, J., MacIntyre, C.R., Mathai, D., 2013. Risk factors for tuberculosis. *Pulm. Med.* 828939. doi: 10.1155/2013/828939.

Nathan, C.F., Hibbs Jr, J.B., 1991. Role of nitric oxide synthesis in macrophage antimicrobial activity. *Curr. Opin. Immunol.* 3(1), 65–70.

Nicholson, S., Bonecini-Almeida, M.D.G., Lapa e Silva, J.R., Nathan, C., Xie, Q.W., Mumford, R., Weidner, J.R., Calaycay, J., Geng, J., Boechat, N., Linhares, C., Rom, W., Ho, J.L., 1996. Inducible nitric oxide synthase in pulmonary alveolar macrophages from patients with tuberculosis. *J. Exp. Med.* 183(5), 2293–2302.

O'Brien, L., Carmichael, J., Lowrie, D.B., Andrew, P.W., 1994. Strains of Mycobacterium tuberculosis differ in susceptibility to reactive nitrogen intermediates in vitro. *Infect. Immun.* 62(11), 5187–5190.

Palomino, J.C., Leão, S.C., Ritacco, V., 2007. Tuberculosis 2007; from basic science to patient care. www.TuberculosisTextbook.com.

Pasqualoto, K.F.M., Ferreira, E.I., 2001. An approach for the rational design of new anti-tuberculosis agents. *Curr. Drug Targets* 2(4), 427–437.

Robitzek, E.H., Selikoff, I.J., 1952. Hydrazine derivatives of isonicotinic acid (Rimifon, Marsilid) in the treatment of active progressive caseous-pneumonic tuberculosis: A preliminary report. *Am. Rev. Tuberc.* 65(4), 402–428.

Russell, D.G., 2001. Mycobacterium tuberculosis: Here today, and here tomorrow. *Nat. Rev. Mol. Cell Biol.* 2(8), 569–578.

Samet, J.M., Eradze, G.R., 2000. Radon and lung cancer risk: Taking stock at the millenium. *Environ. Health Perspect.* 108(Suppl 4), 635–641.

Sarkar, S., Song, Y., Sarkar, S., Kipen, H.M., Laumbach, R.J., Zhang, J., Strickland, P.A.O., Gardner, C.R., Schwander, S., 2012. Suppression of the NF-κB pathway by diesel exhaust particles impairs human antimycobacterial immunity. *J. Immunol.* 188(6), 2778–2793.

Schatz, A., Bugle, E., Waksman, S.A., 1944. Streptomycin, a substance exhibiting antibiotic activity against gram-positive and gram-negative bacteria. *Proc. Soc. Exp. Biol. Med.* 55(1), 66–69.

Sensi, P., 1983. History of the development of rifampin. *Rev. Infect. Dis.* 5(Suppl 3), S402–S406.

Sharpe, W.C., 1931. Artificial pneumothorax in pulmonary tuberculosis. *Can. Med. Assoc. J.* 25(1), 54–57.

Silva, D.R., Mello, F.C.D.Q., Migliori, G.B., 2020. Shortened tuberculosis treatment regimens: What is new? *J. Bras. Pneumol.* 46(2), e20200009. doi: 10.36416/1806-3756/e20200009.

Smith, G.S., Stephen, K., Van, D.E., Cynthia, G., Jun, S., Roger, B., Amy, H.H., David, B.R., Annelies, V.R., Michael, E., Marilie, D.G., 2016. Air pollution and pulmonary tuberculosis: A nested case–control study among members of a northern California health plan. *Environ. Health Perspect.* 124(6), 761–768.

Smith, I., 2003. Mycobacterium tuberculosis pathogenesis and molecular determinants of virulence. *Clin. Microbiol. Rev.* 16(3), 463–496.

Thomas, J.P., Baughn, C.O., Wilkinson, R.G., Shepherd, R.G., 1961. A new synthetic compound with antituberculous activity in mice: Ethambutol (dextro-2, 2′-(ethylenediimino)-di-1-butanol). *Am. Rev. Respir. Dis.* 83(6), 891–893.

Tufariello, J.M., Chan, J., Flynn, J.L., 2003. Latent tuberculosis: Mechanisms of host and bacillus that contribute to persistent infection. *Lancet Infect. Dis.* 3(9), 578–590.

Types of Pollutants - Air Quality and Health. WHO. Available online at https://www.who.int/teams/environment-climate-change-and-health/air-quality-and-health/health-impacts/types-of-pollutants (accessed on July 10, 2022).

Urdahl, K.B., Shafiani, S., Ernst, J.D., 2011. Initiation and regulation of T-cell responses in tuberculosis. *Mucosal Immunol.* 4(3), 288–293.

Volmink, J., Garner, P., 2007. Directly observed therapy for treating tuberculosis. *Cochrane Database Syst. Rev.* 4, CD003343. doi: 10.1002/14651858.CD003343.pub3.

Wei, X.Q., Charles, I.G., Smith, A., Ure, J., Feng, G.J., Huang, F.P., Xu, D., Mullers, W., Moncada, S., Liew, F.Y., 1995. Altered immune responses in mice lacking inducible nitric oxide synthase. *Nature* 375(6530), 408–411.

WHO, 1993. WHO declares tuberculosis a global emergency. *Soz Präventivmed.* 38(4), 251–252.

WHO, 2020. Global tuberculosis report 2020. *Glob. Tuberc. Rep.*, ISBN: 978-92-4-001313-1,232.

WHO, 2021. *Global Tuberculosis Report 2021*. Geneva: World Health Organization.

WHO, *Air Pollution*. WHO. Available online at https://www.who.int/health-topics/air-pollution#tab=tab_1 (accessed on July 8, 2022).

WHO, Stop TB Initiative, 2009. *Treatment of Tuberculosis: Guidelines*, 4th edn. Geneva: World Health Organization.

World Health Organization, 2016. Ambient air pollution: A global assessment of exposure and burden of disease. ISBN: 978924151135,121.

World Health Organization, 2021. WHO global air quality guidelines: Particulate matter (PM2. 5 and PM10), ozone, nitrogen dioxide, sulfur dioxide and carbon monoxide. ISBN: 978924003422,300.

World Health Organization, and Stop TB Initiative (World Health Organization), 2010. *Treatment of Tuberculosis: Guidelines*. Geneva, Switzerland: World Health Organization,

Yang, J., Zhang, M., Chen, Y., Ma, L., Yadikaer, R., Lu, Y., Lou, P., Pu, Y., Xiang, R., Rui, B., 2020. A study on the relationship between air pollution and pulmonary tuberculosis based on the general additive model in Wulumuqi, China. *Int. J. Infect. Dis.* 96, 42–47.

Yang, L., Li, C., Tang, X., 2020. The impact of $PM_{2.5}$ on the host defense of respiratory system. *Front. Cell Dev. Biol.* 8, 91.

Yao, L., LiangLiang, C., JinYue, L., WanMei, S., Lili, S., YiFan, L., HuaiChen, L., 2019. Ambient air pollution exposures and risk of drug-resistant tuberculosis. *Environ. Int.* 124, 161–169.

Zhang, J., Wei, Y., Fang, Z., 2019. Ozone pollution: A major health hazard worldwide. *Front. Immunol.* 10, 2518.

5 Pandemics, Environment, and Globalisation

Understanding the Interlinkage in the Context of COVID-19

Mantosh Kumar Satapathy, Hemant Kumar, Chih-Hao Yang, Ting-Lin Yen, and Papita Das

CONTENTS

5.1 Introduction 63
5.2 Major Pandemics of the 19th, 20th, and 21st Centuries 65
5.2.1 The Flu Pandemic (1889–1890) 65
5.2.2 Spanish Flu (1918–1920) 65
5.2.3 The Asian Flu (1957–1958) 66
5.2.4 AIDS Pandemic and Epidemic (1981–Present) 66
5.2.5 SARS 66
5.2.6 Swine Flu 66
5.2.7 MERS 67
5.2.8 COVID-19 67
5.3 Main Reasons for the Spread of Infectious Diseases 67
5.3.1 Environment and Infectious Diseases 69
5.3.2 Globalisation and Pandemics in the Context of COVID-19 72
5.4 Lessons Learned from Past Pandemics and the Way Forward 73
5.5 Conclusion 76
References 76

5.1 INTRODUCTION

Pathology developing in living organisms due to the entry of microorganisms such as bacteria, viruses, and fungi is known as infectious disease, which may or may not be contagious or emerge as an epidemic or pandemic (Dobson and

DOI: 10.1201/9781003288732-5

Carper, 1996). Since the novel coronavirus disease 2019 (COVID-19) emerged, it has caused the concepts of epidemics, endemics, and pandemics to be revisited (Table 5.1). An epidemic is a condition resulting in a sudden increase in disease cases in a particular geographical region, while an endemic is a disease outbreak consistently present in a specific region, which can be monitored easily (Healthcare, 2020). Conversely, a pandemic is an abruptly growing disease affecting several countries and populations with unexpected exponential spreadability (Morens et al., 2009). Hence, an uncontrolled pandemic crossing the country's geographical boundaries leads to large-scale social disruption, economic loss, and general hardship.

The World Health Organization (WHO) declared COVID-19 a public health emergency of international concern on 30 January 2020, and a pandemic on 11 March 2020 (Adhikari et al., 2020; Tison et al., 2020). The whole world is now facing the new COVID-19 pandemic, an infectious disease caused by the SARS-CoV-2 virus. The current emerging outbreak of COVID-19 necessitates an in-depth investigation into previous infectious diseases, as it is a tremendous public health threat to the world in the 21st century. The crisis facing the world today in the form of COVID-19 is not the first crisis in human history. Human civilisation has faced many such natural and anthropogenic calamities and crises in its development journey. Furthermore, in the context of the current COVID-19, this is not the first time such a dreadful pandemic has hit the world. Previously, cholera, plague, chickenpox, influenza, Spanish flu, Asian flu, the seventh cholera pandemic, Hong Kong flu, severe acute respiratory syndrome (SARS), swine flu, Middle East respiratory syndrome (MERS), human immuno-deficiency virus (HIV)/acquired immune deficiency syndrome (AIDS), tuberculosis (TB), and malaria have severely threatened human life.

TABLE 5.1
Generalised ideas about endemic, epidemic, and pandemic diseases

Disease Type	Characteristics	Example(s)
Endemic	Diseases developing from pathogens that continuously/seasonally affect a particular geographic area or population group and are consistently present in that specific region	Malaria in Nigeria
Epidemic	When there is an unexpected increase in the number of disease cases in a specific geographical area; it may or may not be contagious	Ebola virus disease in East and West Africa, Zika virus disease in the Americas
Pandemic	When an epidemic has spread over multiple countries or continents with wide geographical dispersion, high attack rates and explosiveness, novelty, rapid infectiousness, contagiousness, disease motility, and severity	Spanish flu, swine flu, COVID-19

Following these major pandemics, the recent devastating outbreak of COVID-19 in the 21st century has impelled the scientific community to ask questions for the future, such as the correlation between environmental change and newer infectious pathologies, and globalisation and its impact on global health and the economy during the pandemics. Recent research communication focuses mainly on maintaining ecological stability and global health. Hence, COVID-19 research requires further investigations on how the spread of COVID-19 is interrelated with environmental damage, climate change, and global travel. Additional studies are necessary to analyse these interactions and mechanisms to find effective measures, policies, and research perspectives, as COVID-19 will be a long-lasting global threat. Therefore, this chapter comprehensively focuses on the history of recent major pandemics and the connection between pandemics, ecological imbalance, and globalisation, specifically in the context of COVID-19, which will be a valuable addition to the research regarding pandemic control and environmental sustainability.

5.2 MAJOR PANDEMICS OF THE 19TH, 20TH, AND 21ST CENTURIES

The current COVID-19 outbreak is not the only disease to have impacted the world on a global scale. Some of the major pandemics of history, such as cholera, influenza, and the recent coronavirus disease, have been reviewed globally (Piret and Boivin, 2021). Most studies illustrate that the majority of recent pandemics are due to the spread of the severely contagious influenza virus. Several infectious diseases, including flu, have left deeper footprints in the world history of pandemics (Falode et al., 2021). The contemporary COVID-19 has been shown to surpass the influenza of the past in virulence. Therefore, it is necessary to have a basic understanding of previous pandemics and the multifarious measures used to handle them.

5.2.1 The Flu Pandemic (1889–1890)

The influenza pandemic started in the 18th–19th century, and its effects are still felt throughout the globe. Influenza viruses belong to the single-stranded RNA viruses of the Orthomyxoviridae family (Wright, 2001). Several influenza virus strains have been identified, including A, B, C, and D. Among these, only the influenza A virus has severe pandemic potential, while B may create seasonal epidemics in temperate regions (Curriero et al., 2002). Advancements in transportation were solely responsible for spreading the influenza virus in the US, Russia, Europe, and the rest of the world, killing one million people.

5.2.2 Spanish Flu (1918–1920)

The Spanish flu was another influenza pandemic that started just after World War I in 1918, spreading worldwide, infecting about 500 million people (one-third of the world's population) and resulting in around 50 million deaths within only 2 years; this was the most severe pandemic in history (Martini et al., 2019). The causative organism was the H1N1 virus (Watanabe and Kawaoka, 2011). People of all age groups were severely affected (mortality was especially high in the age group between 20 and 40 years). Without a successful vaccine, pharmaceutical interventions, and antibiotics, this disease remained uncontrollable. Prohibition of public gatherings, isolation, quarantine, maintenance of hygiene, and disinfection measures were employed to check the spread of the pandemic (Rewar et al., 2015).

5.2.3 The Asian Flu (1957–1958)

The Asian flu was caused by a hybrid strain of bird flu virus. It originated in China and became pandemic, rapidly spreading to Singapore in February 1957 and to Hong Kong and the US in April–July 1957, causing 1.1 million deaths worldwide. This Asian flu pandemic returned in 1968 as the 'Hong Kong flu,' killing about three million people (Wever and Van Bergen, 2014).

5.2.4 AIDS Pandemic and Epidemic (1981–Present)

HIV, found in chimpanzees, was identified as the causative organism for AIDS. AIDS had infected more than 35 million people worldwide by the late 20th century. Unfortunately, there were no effective measures to cure this disease for a long period. However, in the 1990s, specific antiviral formulations were developed to enhance the life span and quality of life of HIV-infected patients (Sharp and Hahn, 2011).

5.2.5 SARS

SARS originated in southern China in 2002. It was transmitted from infected bats (palm civets) to humans. Pneumonia, the primary symptom of SARS, was infectious and sometimes fatal. China and Hong Kong were the most severely hit, with 80% of the population affected by SARS. The virus further affected more than 30 countries, and 774 deaths were reported (Lee, 2005; Hung, 2003).

5.2.6 Swine Flu

Swine flu originated in pigs. It started spreading in Mexico in 2009–2010 and was declared a pandemic due to its rapid global spread. This was a respiratory infection caused by the H1N1 virus. The major pathological symptoms are like those of other flus, such as periodic fever, chills, cough, sore throat, runny or stuffy nose, watery red eyes, body aches, and headache. The estimated mortality was between 151,700 and 575,400 (Dawood et al., 2012). Within a few weeks of its onset, the swine flu had spread to more than 30 countries, mainly due to global trade. This flu also had severe adverse socio-economic consequences due to the high mortality rate. Certain antiviral drugs, like Zanamivir and Oseltamivir, and other pharmaceutical and non-pharmaceutical interventions are used for prophylaxis and cure (Rubin et al., 2009).

5.2.7 MERS

MERS was first reported in Saudi Arabia in 2012, caused by the MERS coronavirus (MERS-CoV), a zoonotic virus from infected dromedary camels, spread, and became pandemic. The main pathology in humans is a severe respiratory illness with fever, cough, and shortness of breath. A death toll of 858 was reported in 27 countries, including the Middle East, the US, Africa, South Asia, and others, mostly showing human-to-human transmission (Memish et al., 2020; Kusuma et al., 2021).

5.2.8 COVID-19

The current COVID-19 is an unprecedented and ongoing pandemic, since there is no known cure. Compared with the devastating 'Spanish flu,' which took almost a year to become a global pandemic, COVID-19 became a global pandemic within only 2–3 months. Surpassing Hong Kong flu, Asian flu, and SARS-CoV, SARS-CoV-2 exhibited extraordinary mortality and morbidity globally (Zhang et al., 2020; Al Hasan et al., 2020). The WHO has recorded six million deaths worldwide due to the novel COVID-19 (WHO Coronavirus COVID-19-Dashboard, https://covid19.who.int/). This highly contagious disease is believed to have originated in bats. Human-to-human transmission occurs through inhaling droplets during coughing or sneezing. The major pathological symptoms include fever, cough, shortness of breath, muscle pain, severe pneumonia, sepsis, shock, multiple organ failure, and death. Ageing societies with compromised health (hypertension, diabetes, and chronic respiratory disease) are more susceptible to COVID-19 infection and mortality (Jordan et al., 2020). Due to its severity and rapid spread of infection, in early 2020, the WHO declared the disease a public health emergency of international concern (Zhao et al., 2020). COVID-19 had great socio-economic, political, and technological impact along with public health concerns, resulting in a deep global recession.

The major pandemics of recent centuries are outlined chronologically in Table 5.2.

5.3 MAIN REASONS FOR THE SPREAD OF INFECTIOUS DISEASES

Infectious diseases are caused by microorganisms such as bacteria, viruses, or parasites, which spread from one person to another through various vectors such as humans, other animals, or other organisms. Infectious diseases may further develop into endemics, epidemics, or pandemics. Scientific studies on past

TABLE 5.2
Chronological representation of major pandemics of recent centuries

Period	Pandemic	Pathogen	Vector(s)	Death Toll
1918–1919	Spanish flu	Influenza A/H1N1	Avian	50 million
1957–1959	Asian flu	Influenza A/H2N2	Avian	1 million
1968–1970	Hong Kong flu	Influenza A/H3N2	Avian	1 million
1981–ongoing	Acquired immunodeficiency syndrome (AIDS)	HIV	Humans and other animals	36.3 million
2002–2003	Severe acute respiratory syndrome (SARS)	SARS-CoV	Bats, palm civets	774
2009–2010	Swine flu	Influenza A/H1N1	Pigs	200,000
2015–ongoing	Middle East respiratory syndrome (MERS)	MERS-CoV	Bats, dromedary camels	888
2019–ongoing	COVID-19	SARS-CoV-2	Bats, pangolins	6.02 million

infectious diseases show that several factors are responsible for outbreaks as well as the causative pathogens. Human interactions play a direct or indirect role in spreading infectious diseases (Honigsbaum, 2009). Epidemiology may uncover some related factors behind contagious disease outbreaks (Danon et al., 2011). The various factors responsible for the initial origin of the infectious diseases include new or mutant pathogens, ecological imbalance, nature's response in the form of natural disasters, natural toxins, undetected chemical release, and toxic radiation. These factors also catalyse disease transmission through environmental routes like water, air, and food. Furthermore, increasing globalisation is another major factor responsible for spreading infectious diseases. Here, the interconnectedness of the environment and globalisation is explained in the context of spreading infectious diseases and management to prevent future pandemics such as COVID-19.

5.3.1 Environment and Infectious Diseases

In 2016, the United Nations Environment Programme specified that 75% of all emerging infectious diseases in humans are zoonotic and closely interlinked with environmental health (Everard et al., 2020). The diseases are always present in the environment, remaining suppressed or hidden from human beings. Mother Nature maintains a perfect balance in suppressing pathogenic microorganisms in the environment. However, loss of natural habitat and environmental destruction are responsible for the sudden exposure of hidden pathogenic organisms, with severe health impacts on humans. Biodiversity loss is among the foremost dangers to human health, exposing people worldwide to infectious disease threats (Iacono et al., 2018). Man-made environmental changes are the major driving forces for disease events and infectious disease transmission via biological and ecological processes (Lustgarten, 2020; Lawler et al., 2021). Environmental balance loss is caused by agriculture, industrialisation, urbanisation, deforestation, carbon dioxide, methane, and nitrous oxide. Furthermore, ozone gas emission leads to a sudden change in rainfall, humidity, and climate change, increasing surface temperatures and furthering the emergence of novel pathogens. Moreover, changing ecology brings the animals carrying the pathogenic microorganisms from forests into new areas, increasing the risk of infection (Thomas, 2020; Biota, 2002). In general, zoonotic microorganisms remain inert and stable in an animal reservoir, but spill over to the environment under adverse environmental conditions to develop pathologies in humans, which can then be passed on to other humans. Several examples of past infectious diseases in correlation with the environment and ecological change are presented here. A previous study showed that in 2018, humans were infected by the Hendra virus from horses. The virus had been transmitted from flying foxes due to severe climate change and virus spillover (Jameel, 2020).

Methane and carbon dioxide (about 1.7 trillion tons of carbon) are sealed in permafrost and glaciers. All this carbon could be converted into a carbon sink and further accelerate global warming (Jameel, 2020). Furthermore, melting permafrost could possibly release dormant human pathogens, a growing concern recently. A study found 33 new virus species in two ice core samples (520 and 15,000 years old) in northwestern Tibet, among which 28 were novel (Zhong et al., 2020). One study estimated that more than 3,200 strains of coronaviruses already exist among bats, awaiting an opportunity to jump to people (Lustgarten, 2020). Deforestation is another major cause of severe biodiversity loss, resulting in oxygen level depletion and further aggravating climatic change, leading to the outbreak of infections due to dormant infectious pathogenic microorganisms.

Studies had shown that even before the COVID-19 pandemic, humans throughout the globe had been severely affected by HIV/AIDS, Ebola, MERS, Zika, various flus, and SARS due to changes in environmental factors. For example, the WHO (www.who.int/teams/global-hiv-hepatitis-and-stis-programmes/hiv/strategic-information/hiv-data-and-statistics) recorded approximately 37.7 million HIV-infected people between the 1980s and 2020, with 1.5 million new cases originating from a type of chimpanzee in Central Africa. Further, there may be a direct or indirect connection between HIV/AIDS and the environment responsible for its outbreak. Migration due to climate change also has an important role in spreading HIV, possibly forcing the population to move from a compromised habitat (climate refugees) to a better climatic habitat, where they may be infected due to large sexual networks (Mauambeta, 2003; Ngigi, 2006). Poverty, migration, and depleted economic status due to climate change are all indirect risk factors for HIV transmission; they indirectly affect human health and immunity, favouring disease transmission (Bolton, 2010; Bolton and Talman, 2010).

Ebola virus disease (EVD), primarily found in Africa, is transmitted zoonotically to humans, monkeys, and gorillas from infected avians such as bats (World Health Organization, 2021; Taylor et al., 2001). The major pathological symptom is haemorrhagic fever, often with a high case fatality rate in diagnosed patients (Legrand et al., 2007). This EVD outbreak was caused by four pathogenic strains of Ebola virus: Zaire (EBOV), Sudan (SUDV), Taï Forest (TAFV), and Bundibugyo (BDBV), mainly affecting vulnerable communities with low immunity as a result of migration from one place to another because of sudden environmental changes (Hotez et al., 2009; Grace et al., 2012; Pigott et al., 2014). The changed environment could have activated the dormant pathogens in the environment, infecting the bats, and further humans were infected and acted as spreaders of the disease (Kassie et al., 2015).

The WHO reported that the MERS-CoV infection started in Saudi Arabia in 2012 and spread to 27 countries, including the Middle East, North Africa, Europe, the US, and Asia. The symptoms are mostly like those observed with influenza, severe respiratory tract infection, and pneumonia. People with underlying abnormal health complications such as diabetes, hypertension, and renal failure were at a higher risk of infection and death (World Health Organization, 2019). Environmental factors also contribute to the transmission of the disease. A rise in environmental temperature, high ultraviolet index, low wind speed, and low relative humidity are responsible for spreading this disease (Altamimi and Ahmed, 2020). Initially identified in Ugandan monkeys (1947) infected by a mosquito (*Aedes aegypti*) bearing flavivirus in 1947, the Zika virus disease was later identified in humans in 1952. This deadly virus is transmitted perinatally and through sexual contact, blood transfusion, and organ replacement (Kumar et al., 2021). The general symptoms are fever, rash, headache, joint pain, conjunctivitis, and muscle pain. It remained an epidemic in Yap Island (2007), followed by a large outbreak in French Polynesia in 2013, and became a pandemic in Brazil, the Americas, Africa, and other 86 countries around the world from 2015 onwards (Lowe et al., 2020; www.who.int/news-room/fact-sheets/detail/zika-virus). The direct association between Zika and the environment is that unhygienic water bodies created by heavy rainfall, high humidity, and ecological imbalance favour the breeding of the vector *Aedes aegypti*, further spreading the infection to animals. Directly and indirectly, social and environmental drivers also impact the spread of this disease (Fuller et al., 2017). Preventive and control measures include proper sanitisation to prevent mosquito larval growth, use of mosquito repellent, protection from mosquito bites, etc.

As previously discussed, COVID-19 became a pandemic within a short period, caused by a new coronavirus mutant (SARS-CoV-2). Detailed study of other pandemics in history in terms of their origins, interactions with environment and individuals shows a similar pattern of spread of recent COVID-19 (Sage, 2020; Nuñez et al., 2020). The environmental consequences indirectly associated with the pandemic are mainly due to human activities, whether deliberate or not (Diffenbaugh et al., 2020). Various causes of climatic change may contribute to a higher risk of pandemics. For example, deforestation due to urbanisation, industrialisation, and the need for more land (for agricultural and housing purposes) has remained the prime cause of habitat loss. This forces animals to move from their natural habitat. Infections start at that point when severe and spontaneous climatic changes occur. The dormant microorganisms emerge and infect animals, including humans, and the disease begins to spread. For example, ecological imbalance leads to global warming, displacing animals, modifying pathogen ecology, and increasing host–vector interactions in various ways, resulting in spillover of infections from infected animals to humans. Recent findings showed that COVID-19 happened similarly due to virus transfer from the environment to humans through animals such as bats or snakes. Another environmental factor associated with COVID-19 is air pollution. Areas with poor air quality are more susceptible to COVID-19, and the mortality and morbidity rates are higher due to the increased chance of respiratory tract infection (Ondin, 2021). Another major factor, 'adaptive selection' by infectious pathogens, results in genetic mutation and the emergence of more resistant and infectious pandemic pathogens. Recent scientific studies on COVID-19 revealed the genome mutations of SARS-COV-2 virus results in emergence of various Corona-family viruses of recent years which can smartly escape the host's immune system's surveillance (Priyadarsini et al., 2020).

5.3.2 Globalisation and Pandemics in the Context of COVID-19

Globalisation is the multi-faceted expansion of the ideas, information, technologies, investment, people, goods, services, and capital procedures from one country to another worldwide due to growing cross-border trade interdependence (Staff, 2002). It has been speeding up across both international and intranational geographical borders since the 18th century due to significant improvements in transportation technology. The common driving forces for globalisation are technological revolution, advanced economic value-added traits, political impacts, international cultural exchange, and social, environmental, and natural factors. Globalisation directly or indirectly impacts various sectors, including the healthcare sector (Saker et al., 2004). In one way, recently, globalisation has greatly improved public health conditions. The infant mortality rate has been reduced, and life expectancy has increased significantly, after the introduction of globalisation (Ataöv et al., 2010; Martens et al., 2010).

On the contrary, it has also been a major cause of spreading various infectious diseases. Despite technological and economic advancement, humanity is cursed with pandemics (Lindahl and Grace, 2015), including the outbreak of COVID-19 in the 21st century. The spreadability of infectious diseases flares up with various biological, environmental, and social factors such as changing nature of infectious diseases, economic globalisation, global environmental change, global demographic change, and global technological changes. Some pathogenic microorganisms directly or indirectly spread to humans and other animals via primary and/or secondary hosts. Sometimes, the pathogen remains dormant for a certain duration and is suddenly exposed in a dreadful manner in the environment, spreading in the community and globally. The pathogen may be from soil, air, water, or another environment. Humans, animals, and pets, along with foods, unwittingly transport deadly pathogens worldwide. Therefore, infectious diseases easily become pandemic in a contained globalised world regardless of geographical barriers (Jones et al., 2017, Lim, 2014; Tatem et al., 2006). Millions of people travel internationally each year, according to the World Tourism Organization. It is an interesting fact that within 36 hours (short enough to fall within the incubation period of infectious diseases), one can travel throughout the globe carrying infectious pathogens. Most importantly, the increasing ease of air travel and the development of international trade business have noticeably increased the risk of spreading infectious diseases. Furthermore, dangerous microorganisms can be introduced during maritime transport (Dowell, 2002).

Past pandemics could shed light on how the consequences of global migration have spread pandemics and outbreaks (Tatem et al., 2006). The dreadful SARS disease outbreak in 2003 (Qiu, 2017; Lee, 2004; Syed et al., 2003), the swine flu/influenza pandemic (2009–2010) (Gatherer, 2009), and this 21st-century COVID-19 disease (Zoumpourlis et al., 2020) have made it very clear that international trade and travel cause pathogens to spread more rapidly.

Specifically, in the context of COVID-19, the extreme spread of the disease in the globalised world within a very short period is thought-provoking. The prime cause discovered for the transmission of COVID-19 between healthy countries is rapid and intense international travel as a part of globalisation. This dreadful COVID-19 pandemic, combined with other associated factors such as increased flow of humans, rapid urbanisation on a global platform, population growth, demand for animal protein, poor maintenance of animal husbandry, wildlife exploitation, industrialisation, and international trade and travel, is sweeping across the whole world like a wildfire. The COVID-19 pandemic is a highly significant global threat, causing a very large number of deaths and a deep economic recession worldwide.

Therefore, it can be viewed as bearing similarities to previous pandemics by invasive pathogenic microorganisms transmitted globally during their outbreak. In this regard, a detailed and careful study about the COVID-19 pandemic spread may provide an excellent bird's-eye view and acknowledge a more comprehensive effort towards controlling the current and future pandemics.

The critical point here is that without any common collective regulatory policy, particularly for resilience and restrictions on movement, globalisation is undoubtedly a risk factor in the context of a pandemic crisis (Lucchese and Pianta, 2020; Blum and Neumärker, 2020). Fortunately, there are many positive aspects of globalisation as well as the negative consequences (such as the risk of infectious disease spread), which need to be focused on carefully. Globalisation facilitates faster communication, effective teamwork with better collaboration, and efficient communication, which will facilitate a more comprehensive universal effort toward controlling pandemics in the future (Duarte and Snyder, 2006). How gradual progress in the economy, integrated trade development, global human migration, and interchange of cultural aspects between countries impact the patterns of pandemic emergence needs to be studied. In addition, various policies should be implemented in response to infectious diseases on a scientific basis, supporting contemporary and possible global approaches. Further careful measures and fresh response methods and tools should be introduced into private industry, public health agencies, regulatory agencies, policy makers, academics, and research sectors (Figure 5.1).

5.4 LESSONS LEARNED FROM PAST PANDEMICS AND THE WAY FORWARD

With no cure, COVID-19 is an early warning, calling humanity to prepare for future pandemics. The current pandemic situation is a chance that cannot be missed to set the balance. Inger Andersen, the UN environment chief, once stated: 'We are not taking care of ourselves and our planet. This is the message nature is sending us with the coronavirus pandemic' (Mitra, Andersen and Rockström, 2020). Nature will have the final word, and pandemics are a checkpoint for humanity's aberrant behaviours. There may be more disruptive pandemics yet to come. Although there seems to be no direct connection between biodiversity loss and pandemics, climate and environmental changes in a natural habitat are

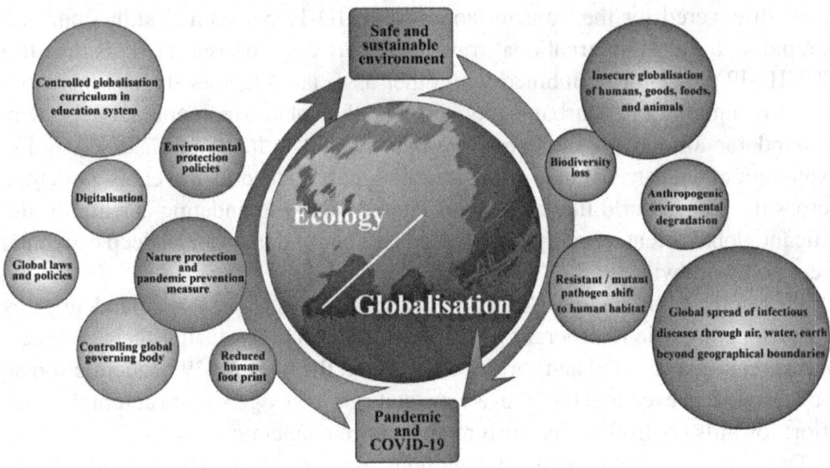

FIGURE 5.1 The interlinkage between the environment and globalisation in the context of the spread and control of infectious diseases.

a warning of the potential jumping of deadly pathogens from the environment to humans through various vectors.

COVID-19 and other pandemics need to be studied further. It is well understood that pandemics and global climate change are closely related. So, targeting the pandemics through various policies that address both would be easier. Furthermore, although globalisation increases the risk of spreading infectious diseases, it also facilitates collaboration and better communication, allowing a more comprehensive global effort towards controlling these diseases. Thus, policies related to climate change and in-depth studies on globalisation seem to be indivisible from efforts to prevent new infectious outbreaks.

Some of the critical points based on the lessons learned from previous pandemics, which could stop the spread of COVID-19 and prevent further pandemics and associated devastation, are presented as follows.

- Human-mediated climate change and biodiversity loss must be checked safely and sustainably. Proper and prompt climate mitigation actions may improve human health, reducing pandemic risks before they spread from natural habitats through vectors. At the same time, interaction with wildlife should be controlled by strictly avoiding human footprints on the shared habitat to restore altered ecosystems. Furthermore, the industrialisation of animal agriculture should be minimised along with less demand for animal meat, as sustainable animal husbandry could decrease greenhouse gas emissions, indirectly reducing the risk of infectious diseases.
- There are many pathogenic microorganisms with different pandemic potential depending on the region, origin, resources, habitat, and other

environmental factors. Therefore, a deep investigation is required to determine their common criteria in order to move forward with effective preparedness and response.

- The wildlife trade is another important part of globalisation and a parameter to be controlled wisely. It plays an important role in the transmission of many viruses and bacteria that can cause global pandemics. Hence, the illegal wildlife trade must be transparently and accountably regulated internationally through international policies.
- Multi-faceted and complex regulatory systems must be introduced with various governing systems and bodies, such as the One Health concept, global policy bodies, communism, and totalitarian political systems. To deal with a situation like the COVID-19 pandemic, all the countries' governments must show political interest at the international level so that cooperative international law can be implemented to control illegal wildlife trade, global warming, and vaccine development and production. Such an international platform must be created to monitor and prevent infectious epidemics before an outbreak. Also, international organisations like the WHO should improve their power and structure to address the COVID-19 pandemic and other disease outbreaks. The WHO has to effectively implement new technologies and products as a part of a combinatorial system of globalisation, which can benefit even the world's developing countries that lack modern health and research infrastructure, and people who are deprived of health services can be provided with affordable and speedy health facilities.
- Information technology (IT) and digitalisation are the most important emerging tools in this modern globalised world. Innovative IT and digitalisation can easily create numerous online apps, websites, and social media networking in various sectors and improve communication. This will enable efficient working even in remote areas during pandemics, such as online working, an online education and healthcare system, online monitoring of disease spread and control, pharmaceutical and non-pharmaceutical intervention measures, vaccination strategies, and online payment methods.
- Pandemic preparedness is the most cost-effective and vital strategy, especially in resource-constrained settings. This could consist of strengthening core public healthcare systems like building and maintenance infrastructure, providing or improving water and sanitation systems, and creating greater awareness. Such measures could rapidly extinguish outbreaks that might otherwise lead to pandemics.

Lastly, sustainable development should be an integral part of all measures taken to prevent, control, and manage present and future pandemics. It is well understood that the environment plays a significant role both in the imbalanced earth and in the modern globalised world, which contributes to the spread of infectious diseases. Consequently, all measures during pandemic control must align with new policies for a sustainable and clean environment, so that pathogenic microbes hidden in the womb of Mother Nature can be prevented from coming into direct contact with humans.

5.5 CONCLUSION

The current COVID-19 crisis and other infectious pandemics necessitate finding links between environmental changes and the emergence of infectious diseases. Diseases in the form of epidemics, endemics, or pandemics or in hidden forms have always existed on this planet. The most interesting fact is that Mother Nature's natural defence systems suppress them. On the contrary, the planet's defence systems fail due to biodiversity loss caused by anthropogenic activities, resulting in the emergence and spread of diseases. Controlling them has proved to be highly challenging in a globalised world. The present COVID-19 pandemic is a warning to set the ecological balance right now. Effective preparedness in the present may prevent and deal with future pandemics. Based on in-depth studies and lessons learned from past pandemics, there may be better preventive measures to manage similar future infectious disease outbreaks in an environmentally sustainable manner. Henceforth, much could be done in terms of the "Pandemic Prevention Initiative" with global networking of non-profit international organizations, inter-government policy making bodies, research laboratories, and private companies to implement strict regulation that can protect the globe from new and emerging pandemics. Furthermore, introducing COVID-19 training courses in the curriculum can create awareness in minimising future pandemic spread.

REFERENCES

Adhikari, Sasmita Poudel, Sha Meng, Yu-Ju Wu, Yu-Ping Mao, Rui-Xue Ye, Qing-Zhi Wang, Chang Sun, Sean Sylvia, Scott Rozelle, and Hein Raat. 2020. "Epidemiology, causes, clinical manifestation and diagnosis, prevention and control of coronavirus disease (COVID-19) during the early outbreak period: A scoping review." *Infectious Diseases of Poverty* 9(1):1–12.

Al Hasan, SM, J Saulam, K Kanda, and T Hirao. 2020. "The novel coronavirus disease (COVID-19) outbreak trends in mainland China: A joinpoint regression analysis of the outbreak data from Jan 10 to Feb 11, 2020." *Bulletin of the World Health Organization* 17. DOI: 10.2471/BLT.20.253153

Altamimi, Asmaa, and Anwar E Ahmed. 2020. "Climate factors and incidence of Middle East respiratory syndrome coronavirus." *Journal of Infection and Public Health* 13(5):704–708.

Andersen, Inger, and J Rockström. 2020. "COVID-19 is a symptom of a bigger problem: Our planet's ailing health." *Time.com, Diakses* 12. https://time.com/5848681/covid-19-world-environment-day/

Ataöv, Anli, Benedicte Brøgger, and Jarle Moss Hildrum. 2010. "An action research approach to the inclusion of immigrants in work life and local community life: Preparation of a participatory realm." *Action Research* 8(3):237–265.

Biota, Marine. 2002. "Climate warming and disease risks for terrestrial." *Science* 1063699(2158):296.

Blum, Bianca, and Bernhard Neumärker. 2020. "Globalization, environmental damage and the corona pandemic-lessons from the crisis for economic, environmental and social policy." *Environmental and Social Policy.* doi:10.13140/RG.2.2.10599.68008

Bolton, Susan, and Anna Talman. 2010. "Interactions between HIV/AIDS and the environment." *A Review of the Evidence and Recommendations for Next Steps: IUCN-ESARO Office, Nairobi, Kenya.*

Bolton, Susan M. 2010. *"Interactions between HIV/AIDS and the environment: A review of the evidence and recommendations for next steps."*Nairobi, Kenya: IUCN ESARO Office. viii + 62pp . URI: http://hdl.handle.net/10625/45317.

Curriero, Frank C, Karlyn S Heiner, Jonathan M Samet, Scott L Zeger, Lisa Strug, and Jonathan A Patz. 2002. "Temperature and mortality in 11 cities of the eastern United States." *American Journal of Epidemiology* 155(1):80–87.

Danon, Leon, Ashley P Ford, Thomas House, Chris P Jewell, Matt J Keeling, Gareth O Roberts, Joshua V Ross, and Matthew C Vernon. 2011. "Networks and the epidemiology of infectious disease." *Interdisciplinary Perspectives on Infectious Diseases* 2011: 28. https://doi.org/10.1155/2011/284909

Dawood, Fatimah S, A Danielle Iuliano, Carrie Reed, Martin I Meltzer, David K Shay, Po-Yung Cheng, Don Bandaranayake, Robert F Breiman, W Abdullah Brooks, and Philippe Buchy. 2012. "Estimated global mortality associated with the first 12 months of 2009 pandemic influenza A H1N1 virus circulation: A modelling study." *The Lancet Infectious Diseases* 12(9):687–695.

Diffenbaugh, Noah S, Christopher B Field, Eric A Appel, Ines L Azevedo, Dennis D Baldocchi, Marshall Burke, Jennifer A Burney, Philippe Ciais, Steven J Davis, and Arlene M Fiore. 2020. "The COVID-19 lockdowns: A window into the earth system." *Nature Reviews Earth and Environment* 1(9):470–481.

Dobson, Andrew P, and E Robin Carper. 1996. "Infectious diseases and human population history." *Bio-Science* 46(2):115–126.

Dowell, Scott F. 2002. *Protecting the Nation's Health in an Era of Globalization: CDC's Global Infectious Disease Strategy: Department of Health and Human Services.* Atlanta: Centers for Disease Control.

Duarte, Deborah L, and Nancy Tennant Snyder. 2006. *Mastering Virtual Teams: Strategies, Tools, and Techniques That Succeed.* John Wiley & Sons.ISBN: 978-0-787-98280-5

Everard, Mark, Paul Johnston, David Santillo, and Chad Staddon. 2020. "The role of ecosystems in mitigation and management of Covid-19 and other zoonoses." *Environmental Science and Policy* 111:7–17.

Falode, Adewunmi James, Joshua Olusegun Bolarinwa, and Moses Yakubu. 2021. "History of pandemics in the twentieth and twenty-first century." *Synesis: Journal of Humanities and Social Sciences* 2(1):9–26.

Fuller, Trevon, Guilherme A Calvet, Camila Genaro Estevam, Patricia Brasil, Jussara Rafael Angelo, Thomas B Smith, and Ana M Bispo Di Filippis. 2017. "Environmental and climatic risk factors for Zika and Chikungunya virus infections in Rio de Janeiro, Brazil, 2015–2016." *Open Forum Infectious Diseases* 4(1): S56.

Gatherer, Derek. 2009. "The 2009 H1N1 influenza outbreak in its historical context." *Journal of Clinical Virology* 45(3):174–178.

Grace, Delia, F Mutua, P Ochungo, RL Kruska, K Jones, L Brierley, Ma Lapar, Mohammed Yahya Said, Mario T Herrero, and PM Phuc. 2012. "Mapping of poverty and likely zoonoses hotspots." Zoonoses Project 4. Report to the UK Department for International Development. Nairobi, Kenya: ILRI. https://hdl.handle.net/10568/21161

Honigsbaum, Mark. 2009. "Pandemic." *The Lancet* 373(9679):1939.

Hotez, Peter J, Alan Fenwick, Lorenzo Savioli, and David H Molyneux. 2009. "Rescuing the bottom billion through control of neglected tropical diseases." *The Lancet* 373(9674):1570–1575.

Hung, Lee Shiu. 2003. "The SARS epidemic in Hong Kong: What lessons have we learned?" *Journal of the Royal Society of Medicine* 96(8):374–378.

Iacono, Giovanni Lo, Andrew A Cunningham, Bernard Bett, Delia Grace, David W Redding, and James LN Wood. 2018. "Environmental limits of Rift Valley fever revealed using ecoepidemiological mechanistic models." *Proceedings of the National Academy of Sciences of the United States of America* 115(31):E7448–E7456.

IMF Staff. 2002. *Globalization: A Framework for IMF Involvement*. Washington, DC: IMF.

Intermountain Healthcare. 2020. "What's the difference between a pandemic, an epidemic, endemic, and an outbreak?" *Intermountainhealthcare.org*.

Jameel, Shahid. 2020. "On ecology and environment as drivers of human disease and pandemics.", ORF Issue Brief No. 388, July 2020, Observer Research Foundation. https://www.orfonline.org/research/on-ecology-and-environment-as-drivers-of-human-disease-and-pandemics/

Jones, Bryony A, Martha Betson, and Dirk U Pfeiffer. 2017. "Eco-social processes influencing infectious disease emergence and spread." *Parasitology* 144(1):26–36.

Jordan, Rachel E, Peymane Adab, and KK Cheng. 2020. "Covid-19: Risk factors for severe disease and death." *British Medical Journal* 368: m1198. doi:10.1136/bmj.m1198

Kassie, Daouda, Mathieu Bourgarel, and François Roger. 2015. "Climate change and Ebola outbreaks: Are they connected? Our Common Future under Climate Change." Paris, France, CFCC15: 707–708

Kumar, Swatantra, Rajni Nyodu, Vimal K Maurya, and Shailendra K Saxena. 2021. "Zika virus disease: Progress and prospects." In Wollaton, Nottingham, Shamim I. Ahmad (Eds.) *Human Viruses: Diseases, Treatments and Vaccines*, 223–232. Switzerland AG: Springer.

Kusuma, Kandati, Pandeeti Emmanuel Vijay Paul, and Buddolla Viswanath. 2021. "Middle East respiratory syndrome: Outbreak response priorities, treatment strategies, and clinical management approaches." In Buddolla Viswanath (Ed.) *Pandemic Outbreaks in the 21st Century*, 111–122. Academic Press. https://www.sciencedirect.com/book/9780323856621/pandemic-outbreaks-in-the-21st-century#book-description

Lawler, Odette K, Hannah L Allan, Peter WJ Baxter, Romi Castagnino, Marina Corella Tor, Leah E Dann, Joshua Hungerford, Dibesh Karmacharya, Thomas J Lloyd, and María José López-Jara. 2021. "The COVID-19 pandemic is intricately linked to biodiversity loss and ecosystem health." *The Lancet Planetary Health* 5(11):e840–e850.

Lee, Kelley. 2004. "Globalisation: What is it and how does it affect health?" *Medical Journal of Australia* 180(4):156–158.

Lee, SH. 2005. "The SARS epidemic in Hong Kong–a human calamity in the 21st century." *Methods of Information in Medicine* 44(2):293–298.

Legrand, Judith, Rebecca Freeman Grais, Pierre-Yves Boelle, Alain-Jacques Valleron, and Antoine Flahault. 2007. "Understanding the dynamics of Ebola epidemics." *Epidemiology and Infection* 135(4):610–621.

Lim, Poh Lian. 2014. *Travel and the Globalization of Emerging Infections*. Oxford: Oxford University Press.

Lindahl, Johanna F, and Delia Grace. 2015. "The consequences of human actions on risks for infectious diseases: A review." *Infection Ecology and Epidemiology* 5(1):30048.

Lowe, Rachel, Sadie J Ryan, Roché Mahon, Cedric J Van Meerbeeck, Adrian R Trotman, Laura-Lee G Boodram, Mercy J Borbor-Cordova, and Anna M Stewart-Ibarra. 2020. "Building resilience to mosquito-borne diseases in the Caribbean." *Plos Biology* 18(11):e3000791.

Lucchese, Matteo, and Mario Pianta. 2020. “The coming coronavirus crisis: What can we learn?” *Intereconomics* 55(2):98–104.

Lustgarten, Abrahm. 2020. “How climate change is contributing to skyrocketing rates of infectious disease.” *Pro-Publica*, May 7.https://features.propublica.org/climate-migration/model-how-climate-refugees-move-across-continents/

Martens, Pim, Su-Mia Akin, Huynen Maud, and Raza Mohsin. 2010. “Is globalization healthy: A statistical indicator analysis of the impacts of globalization on health.” *Globalization and Health* 6(1):1–14.

Martini, Mariano, Valentina Gazzaniga, Nicola Luigi Bragazzi, and Ilaria Barberis. 2019. “The Spanish influenza Pandemic: A lesson from history 100 years after 1918.” *Journal of Preventive Medicine and Hygiene* 60(1):E64.

Mauambeta, Daulos DC. 2003. “HIV/AIDS mainstreaming in conservation: The case of wildlife and environmental society of Malawi.” Imbe, Malawi: Wildlife and Environmental Society of Malawi.

Memish, Ziad A, Stanley Perlman, Maria D Van Kerkhove, and Alimuddin Zumla. 2020. “Middle East respiratory syndrome.” *The Lancet* 395(10229):1063–1077.

Mitra, Vidhi. “Environment and COVID-19: Lessons learned the hard way.” https://legalaiddnlu.wordpress.com/2020/07/02/environment-and-covid-19-lessons-learned-the-hard-way/

Morens, David M, Gregory K Folkers, and Anthony S Fauci. 2009. “What is a pandemic?” *The Journal of Infectious Diseases* 200(7):1018–1021.

Ngigi, MM. 2006. “A geographical study on the HIV/AIDS pandemic in Kenya, Tsukuba.” Ph. D. Dissertation. University of Tsukuba.

Nuñez, Martin A, Anibal Pauchard, and Anthony Ricciardi. 2020. “Invasion science and the global spread of SARS-CoV-2.” *Trends in Ecology and Evolution* 35(8):642–645.

Ondin, Bekir Sitki. 2021. “A view of what pandemic itself tells us in terms of climate change and what it made complex.” SocArXiv j7ebm, Center for Open Science. December 8 DOI: 10.31219/osf.io/j7ebm

Pigott, David M, Nick Golding, Adrian Mylne, Zhi Huang, Andrew J Henry, Daniel J Weiss, Oliver J Brady, Moritz UG Kraemer, David L Smith, and Catherine L Moyes. 2014. “Mapping the zoonotic niche of Ebola virus disease in Africa.” *eLife* 3:e04395.

Piret, Jocelyne, and Guy Boivin. 2021. “Pandemics throughout history.” *Frontiers in Microbiology* 11: 631736.

Priyadarsini, S Lakshmi, M Suresh, and Donald Huisingh. 2020. “What can we learn from previous pandemics to reduce the frequency of emerging infectious diseases like COVID-19?” *Global Transitions* 2:202–220.

Qiu, Jane. 2017. “One world, one health: Combating infectious diseases in the age of globalization.” *National Science Review* 4(3):493–499.

Rewar, Suresh, Dashrath Mirdha, and Prahlad Rewar. 2015. “Treatment and prevention of pandemic H1N1 influenza.” *Annals of Global Health* 81(5):645–653.

Rubin, G James, Richard Amlôt, Lisa Page, and Simon Wessely. 2009. “Public perceptions, anxiety, and behaviour change in relation to the swine flu outbreak: Cross sectional telephone survey.” *BMJ: British Medical Journal* 339. b2651 doi:10.1136/bmj.b2651

Sage, Rowan F. 2020. “Global change biology: A primer.” *Global Change Biology* 26(1):3–30.

Saker, Lance, Kelley Lee, Barbara Cannito, Anna Gilmore, and Diarmid H Campbell-Lendrum. 2004. “Globalization and infectious diseases: A review of the linkages.” World Health Organization. https://apps.who.int/iris/handle/10665/68726

Sharp, Paul M, and Beatrice H Hahn. 2011. “Origins of HIV and the AIDS pandemic.” *Cold Spring Harbor Perspectives in Medicine* 1(1):a006841.

Syed, Qutub, Will Sopwith, Martyn Regan, and Mark A Bellis. 2003. "Behind the mask. Journey through an epidemic: Some observations of contrasting public health responses to SARS." *Journal of Epidemiology and Community Health* 57(11):855–856.

Tatem, Andrew J, David J Rogers, and Simon I Hay. 2006. "Global transport networks and infectious disease spread." *Advances in Parasitology* 62:293–343.

Taylor, Louise H, Sophia M Latham, and Mark EJ Woolhouse. 2001. "Risk factors for human disease emergence." *Philosophical Transactions of the Royal Society of London. Series B: Biological Sciences* 356(1411):983–989.

Thomas, Matthew B. 2020. *Epidemics on the Move: Climate Change and Infectious Disease*. Public Library of Science San Francisco.

Tison, Geoffrey H, Robert Avram, Peter Kuhar, Sean Abreau, Greg M Marcus, Mark J Pletcher, and Jeffrey E Olgin. 2020. "Worldwide effect of COVID-19 on physical activity: A descriptive study." *Annals of Internal Medicine* 173(9):767–770.

Watanabe, Tokiko, and Yoshihiro Kawaoka. 2011. "Pathogenesis of the 1918 pandemic influenza virus." *PLOS Pathogens* 7(1):e1001218.

Wever, Peter C, and Leo Van Bergen. 2014. "Death from 1918 pandemic influenza during the first world war: A perspective from personal and anecdotal evidence." *Influenza and Other Respiratory Viruses* 8(5):538–546.

World Health Organization. 2018. "WHO MERS global summary and assessment of risk." August 2018 [cited 2019 June 5].

World Health Organization. 2019. "WHO MERS global summary and assessment of risk." July 2019, World Health Organization.

World Health Organization. 2021. "Weekly bulletin on outbreak and other emergencies: Week 43: October 18–24, 2021."

Wright, Peter F. 2001. "Orthomyxoviruses." In: Fields, B.N. and Knipe, D.M. Eds., *Fields Virology.* , 4th Edition, Philadelphia: Lippincott Williams & Wilkins, 1533–1579.

Zhang, Yan, Meng Xiao, Shulan Zhang, Peng Xia, Wei Cao, Wei Jiang, Huan Chen, Xin Ding, Hua Zhao, and Hongmin Zhang. 2020. "Coagulopathy and antiphospholipid antibodies in patients with Covid-19." *New England Journal of Medicine* 382(17):e38.

Zhao, Siya, Jin Cao, Qianling Shi, Zijun Wang, Janne Estill, Shuya Lu, Xufei Luo, Junxian Zhao, Hairong Zhang, and Jianjian Wang. 2020. "A quality evaluation of guidelines on five different viruses causing public health emergencies of international concern." *Annals of Translational Medicine* 8(7): 500.

Zhong, Zhi-Ping, Natalie E Solonenko, Yueh-Fen Li, Maria C Gazitúa, Simon Roux, Mary E Davis, James L Van Etten, Ellen Mosley-Thompson, Virginia I Rich, and Matthew B Sullivan. 2020. "Glacier ice archives fifteen-thousand-year-old viruses." *BioRxiv* 2020: 2020.

Zoumpourlis, Vassilios, Maria Goulielmaki, Emmanouil Rizos, Stella Baliou, and Demetrios A Spandidos. 2020. "[Comment]. The COVID19 pandemic as a scientific and social challenge in the 21st century." *Molecular Medicine Reports* 22(4):3035–3048.

6 Climate Change and Zoonotic Diseases

Malaria, Plague, Dengue, and Encephalitis

Raj Kishor Pandey, Amit Kumar Dubey, Simran Sharma, and Chitra Rani

CONTENTS

6.1 Introduction 82
6.2 Malaria: Impact of Climate Change 83
 6.2.1 Global Scenario: Disease, Prevention, and Therapeutics 83
 6.2.2 Climatic Factors: Linkages Between Environment and Malaria Transmission 83
 6.2.3 Predictive Model: Forecast Future Climatic Influences on Malaria 84
 6.2.4 Case Studies: Analysing Seasonal Variations and Malaria Transmission 84
 6.2.5 Newer Modalities: Prediction Methods 85
6.3 Plague: Impact of Climate Change 85
 6.3.1 Global Scenario: Disease, Prevention, and Therapeutics 85
 6.3.2 Climatic Factors: Linkages Between Environment and Plague Transmission 86
 6.3.3 Predictive Modelling: Forecast Future Climatic Influences on Plague 87
 6.3.4 Case Studies: Analysing Seasonal Variations and Plague Transmission 87
 6.3.5 Newer Modalities: Prediction Methods 88
6.4 Dengue 88
 6.4.1 Introduction 88
 6.4.2 Dengue Vector Ecology and Distribution 89
 6.4.3 Impact of Climatic Factors on Dengue 89
 6.4.4 Prevention and Treatment 90
6.5 Encephalitis 90
 6.5.1 Background 90

DOI: 10.1201/9781003288732-6

6.5.2 Ecological Parameters and Climatic Factors Associated with Encephalitis Transmission 91
6.5.3 Vaccination and Therapeutic Approach to Encephalitis 92
6.6 Conclusion and Remarks 92
References 93

6.1 INTRODUCTION

In the late 19th century, humans discovered that environmental factors and geo-relocation of vectors exert an influence on epidemic diseases (Oliveria et al., 2016). Any gradual changes in the transmission pattern/species shift are most likely due to the outcome of climatic changes. Infectious diseases and climatic shifts are interrelated. Climatic conditions significantly aid pandemic progression. Here, we elaborate on the linkage of environmental changes with zoonotic diseases. According to the World Health Organization (WHO), a zoonosis is an infectious disease transmitted via vertebrates to *Homo sapiens*. The reported mortality from zoonoses is ~700,000 cases per year (Joint WHO/FAO Expert Committee, 1959; WHO, 2020). The spread of zoonoses is linked with animals and their transmission vectors (Schaechter, 2012; De Giusti et al., 2019; Leal Filho et al., 2022). These disease carriers may be either mechanical or biological. Globally, the greater the degree or extent of interaction between host and parasites, the greater the progression of the disease (Magouras et al., 2020).

At present, more than 60% of infections are zoonoses (Taylor et al., 2001). Many of these catastrophic infections emerged due to close interactions between humans and rapidly changing climatic conditions. Most of these changes emerge due to natural and man-made disasters. Opportunistic zoonosis affects socio-economic management in the health sector (Fauci et al., 2012). Studies have proven that the emergence or diversification of the zoonoses malaria, plague, dengue, and encephalitis is driven by climatic conditions, and thus leads to disease burden at the global level. Earlier, it was also admitted by humans that adverse climate alterations lead to better adaptation of zoonoses (Health, Human, and National Research Council, 2001). Solar energy shifts that happen because of minor variations in the earth's orbit are a major factor responsible for climate alteration (Rupasinghe et al., 2022). Other factors include global warming, deforestation, urbanisation, globalisation, international trade, etc. (Figure 6.1) (Skea et al., 2021).

The morphological and genomic alteration of transmission carriers (vectors) is also one of the prime factors that helps vectors to remain alive and reproduce in the most favourable environmental conditions: higher temperature and precipitation, etc. It has been observed that with a shift in the elevation and duration of warmer weather, the breeding sites may also shift and thus lead to the diversification of zoonoses.

Therefore, the interlinkage of weather transformation and a shift in the transmission of zoonoses needs to be well understood. This will help in managing the four major zoonotic diseases (malaria, plague, dengue, and encephalitis) and reducing the burden of these diseases.

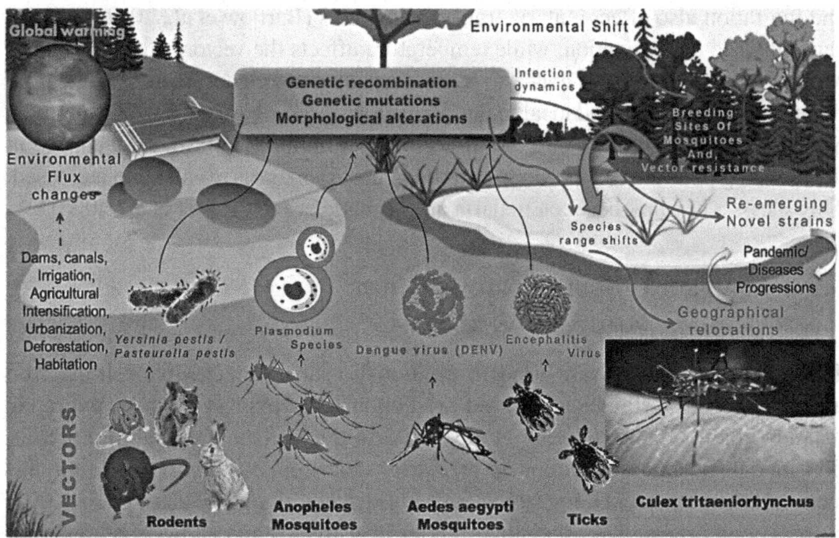

FIGURE 6.1 Schematic illustration of climate changes and zoonotic diseases: plague, malaria, dengue, and encephalitis.

6.2 MALARIA: IMPACT OF CLIMATE CHANGE

6.2.1 Global Scenario: Disease, Prevention, and Therapeutics

Malaria is a type of infectious disease (parasitic) mainly transmitted via the vector, Anopheline mosquitoes. This zoonotic parasitic disease spreads through the bites of infected female mosquitoes (*Anopheles*). The malaria parasite belongs to the *Plasmodium* genus, including five zoonotic forms: *P. falciparum*, *P. vivax*, *P. ovale*, *P. malariae*, and *P. knowlesi.*

> According to the WHO, 219 million malaria cases and 400,000 deaths are reported per year on the global stage (Trottier et al., 2021). The only preventive measures are vector control and anti-malarial drugs (there are no approved vaccines). Mosquirix™ (RTS, S/AS01) is the only vaccine that is approved by WHO and UNICEF specifically for paediatric patients (PATH's Malaria Vaccine Initiative, 2019). The surveillance factors include insecticide-treated nets and in-house anti-malarial spraying.

6.2.2 Climatic Factors: Linkages Between Environment and Malaria Transmission

The question arises: why are there so many cases of malaria? Alterations in the natural climate of a region, which may be either sudden or prolonged, are leading to the prevalence of diseases that were previously rare or of unknown nature. Weather conditions change pathogens and/or disease vehicles to develop and disseminate newer adaptation mechanisms (Huber et al., 2020). Moreover, climatic disasters and migration also affect malaria transmission rates (Bartlow et al., 2019). Rainfall can influence dissemination, while temperature affects the vectors' growth pattern. Malaria, as a public health concern, is most sensitive to long-term atmospheric conditions. On both global and local scales, irrigation systems have changed the periodic nature of malaria episodes and epidemics. Higher humidity influenced a change in the breeding pattern of mosquitoes, and thus, cases of malaria re-infection increased. This shows a key link between malaria and climatic events (Keiser et al., 2005).

6.2.3 Predictive Model: Forecast Future Climatic Influences on Malaria

Three types of models are used to predict the subsequent climatic impact on malarial diseases: statistically based predictions, process based, and topography (islands/inlands) based (Corder et al., 2019). In the statistical probability prediction model, an interconnection is primarily determined by empirical data collection through present geographic zones of disease and particular zone-specific climatic conditions. This statistical model investigates and shows the effects of the climate and human interference on prevalence of disease. The actual transmission of parasitic diseases (vector-borne) can be accurately determined by applying an empirical equation to future weather and assuming negligible human involvement in climatic areas. This type of model has been mostly used in the analysis of malaria behaviour due to climatic influence.

The process-based model is used when parasitologists determine the correlation between weather variables and biological factors (reservoir-to-host disease carrier species' breeding sites, vector growth, sometimes biting rates and incubation times, etc.). It is purely a mathematical model based on a set of equations and is simply applied to gain information regarding vector–parasite transmission. It also indicates that when climatic conditions are transformed, the transmission of malaria (vector) is also affected. This may be combined with human involvement. It has been observed that a small rise in temperature (~2–3 ûC) may push the vectors into zoonotic overflow. There is an increase of about 3–5% (~225 million) in malarial cases, and thus, the seasonal period of malaria expands, and the disease emerges as endemic (Parham et al., 2010).

Lastly, the landscape-based model is used to predict or estimate the effect of climatic conditions on disease carrier habitats (natural terrain). Ground-based and remote sensing techniques are used in this modelling (for different vegetation types/habitats). This has been widely used in African geolocations to understand malarial patterns.

6.2.4 Case Studies: Analysing Seasonal Variations and Malaria Transmission

Several studies have been conducted worldwide to examine the impact of weather/climatic conditions on malaria. The connection of malaria transmission with temperature and precipitation was well described in southern Europe. It was predicted in a study conducted in Portugal that the transmission of malaria into neo-geolocations or prolonged infection time may be possible due to climatic variations (Casimiro et al., 2006). A study in the UK suggested that medium/ moderate increases in weather conditions are the best fit for *P. vivax* species. It was observed that the southeastern part of the UK is more susceptible to malaria transmission (Lindsay et al., 2010). A team of researchers predicted that future climatic conditions will be suitable or the best fit for *Plasmodium* transmission (or vector breeding) in the highland belt of the tropical zones (East Africa) (Caminade et al., 2014).

6.2.5 Newer Modalities: Prediction Methods

New study models implemented in recent years have been found to be effective in estimating climatic changes and geographical areas suitable for malarial transmission. These hydrological and flood models predict the earliest possible emergence of habitats for *Anopheles* mosquitoes or malarial transmission (Smith et al., 2020). A continental-scale hydrological model predicted the hydro-climatic suitability and focal points of malaria transmission at the river corridors. Through that model analysis, performed in South Africa, it was estimated that rather than focusing on eastern areas, it will be more fruitful to focus on the Caledon and Orange rivers, which share a border with Namibia. In South Sudan, it was predicted that in the near future, malaria suitability will decline gradually, as projected by the hydrological approach model. Most of the countries that are vulnerable to malaria have experienced a behavioural change in transmission due to seasonal variations (environmental covariates/ vegetation variance, etc.).

All these studies suggested that climate change or seasonal variations affect the global spread of *Plasmodium* species. Three factors are closely associated: climatic factors, zoonotic malaria, and impact on public health. These statistical and observational studies suggested that a mean rise in temperature would lead to an increasing malaria death rate globally. Therefore, preventive measures have to be established before the disease becomes epidemic. The empirical relationships must be scaled up, and biological phenomena must be well understood with respect to the global/local climatic scenario.

6.3 PLAGUE: IMPACT OF CLIMATE CHANGE

6.3.1 Global Scenario: Disease, Prevention, and Therapeutics

Plague is a rodent-borne zoonosis caused by *Yersinia pestis* (a bacterium). The infection is transmitted to humans from sick rodents (reservoirs: mice, rats, squirrels, etc.) that are infected with fleas, and through flea bites. This is the oldest disease known, also referred to as the Black Death in ancient times. The most common form is bubonic plague. Symptoms include fever, delirium, and the formation of buboes (swollen lymph nodes), the most severe leaking pus. Other plagues are termed septicaemic and pneumonic plague (lung infection) (WHO, 2022; Cleveland Clinic report on Plague, 2021).

At present,, there is no registered vaccine, but therapeutics include antibiotics such as ciprofloxacin, levofloxacin, moxifloxacin (quinolones), gentamicin injection (aminoglycosides), doxycycline (tetracyclines), etc. If treatment is not timely, the fatality rate will be higher. Treatment modalities have to be implemented within 1 week for bubonic plague and within 2 days for pneumonic plague (Demeure et al., 2019). Suggested prevention includes the use of insect repellents, such as DEET/permethrin, for avoiding infected fleas, and avoiding direct contact with pneumonic plague patients.

6.3.2 Climatic Factors: Linkages Between Environment and Plague Transmission

The zoonosis plague (an enzootic cycle) is mostly found in rural/semi-rural regions (semi-arid forestation), grasslands, and woody vegetation areas because these realms have habitats for rodents, such as squirrels, chipmunks, forest rats, voles, and hares, respectively. These rodents are vulnerable and can be easily infected by *Yersinia pestis* (the vector is *Xenopsylla cheopis*). Rodents (order: Rodentia) and fleas (order: Siphonaptera) are long-term reservoirs for *Y. pestis* (Martinez et al., 2018; Demeure et al., 2019). The probability of epizootic cases in humans is greater in the course of cooler summers in the South-West zone of the US because the rodent reservoir density becomes higher in this geographical area due to seasonal shift (wet winter to cooler summer). A single reservoir can extend the infection to diverse habitats.

Therefore, climatic and seasonal variations have a significant impact on rodent breeding. Moreover, the warm climate during the spring season is also favourable for rodent populations, and increased interaction with humans is observed in this time span. This will enhance the probability of plague transmission between the reservoir and the host (Plague – Annual Epidemiological Report, 2021). Further, humid conditions (rainy season) are also favourable for rodent breeding, because heavy rainfall promotes crops, grasses, and herbs, and thus, the rodent population and the rate of interaction with humans increase.

Warm, moist weather is highly suitable for the development, survival, metamorphosis, and behaviour of fleas (*Xenopsylla cheopis*) (Krasnov et al., 2001; Krasnov et al., 2002). Thus, the primary vector of the plague is regulated by temperature change and relative humidity. Being ectothermic, these plague-causing fleas' survival stages are influenced by humid conditions, because low humidity/moisture or high temperature decreases the development of the body mass index (Gage et al., 2008). The larval stage is sensitive to desiccation and depends on adult excreta. Soil moisture is also a controlling factor in the survival of flea larvae (immature stages); this is regulated by optimum precipitation quantity in the soil near rodent burrows (Eisen et al., 2009). However, high organic mass and relative humidity (~95% or more) may also influence fungal growth in nearby rodents' burrows, and thus, flea (*X. cheopis*) larval and/or egg survival are also affected (Parmenter et al., 1999).

Hence, the survival or transmission of *Y. pestis* notably depends on vector or reservoir population, seasonality and geographical zone shifting, etc.

6.3.3 Predictive Modelling: Forecast Future Climatic Influences on Plague

The seasonal variations in a particular geographical area directly affect the distribution of infectious diseases. Pathogens causing zoonoses are vulnerable to meteorological variables (temperature and humidity) because these factors modulate the vector dynamics and bacterial transmission (Eisen et al., 2011).

Models based on estimation of physical parameters (ground-based meteorological data), such as forecasting temperature, precipitation quantity, wind velocity, the density of clouds, etc., and association between climatic conditions, human interaction, and pathogen occurrence may help in determining disease transmission and reduce the disease burden (Patz et al., 2005). Two main types of forecast modelling have been applied in plague disease investigation: local meteorological datasets, and datasets obtained from satellites (gridded climate datasets) where complex topography is present.

There are limitations to meteorological data collection; sometimes, accuracy varies because of selection of undependable variables and the functional interrelation established between physical variables and disease progression. These in-situ data collection and algorithm speculations have some restrictions, as they may not cover the whole range of probable weather outcomes, and thus, disease transmission prediction may vary. This happens mainly in tropical regions (Gage et al., 2008; Gneiting et al., 2005). Therefore, when forecasting disease progression, to get accurate data, satellite-derived and spatial weather-reanalysis image datasets are advanced techniques that can be helpful in obtaining linkage (corelation) between climate and prediction in plague-prone geographical areas.

6.3.4 Case Studies: Analysing Seasonal Variations and Plague Transmission

In a literature survey, various teams postulated a correlation between environmental changes and plague. The emission of greenhouse gases (CO_2, methane) leads to shifting in reservoir populations. Predictive data obtained from Central Asia (Kazakhstan) on plague intensity suggested that even the 1 °C rise in atmospheric temperature in the spring season may result in more than 50% increase of pathogen (*Yersinia pestis*) presence in the host (Stenseth et al., 2006). One specific study in California proposed that climatic alterations may put the human population at risk of infection. The human population in the Sierra Nevada and Northern California coastal regions was found to be more prone to infection. However, lower risk was observed in the south belt of California (Holt et al.,

2009). One more predictive study on plague transmission to newer geolocations was performed, and it was observed that in the coming decades, the plague will shift to higher latitudes (geographic coordinates) and high altitude (far from sea level) rather than western parts of the US (Ari et al., 2010). Another study by Nakazawa and co-workers estimated that there will be zoonotic (plague) shifts in the northward direction/ to the northern latitudes of the US before the year 2060. This will lead to more hotspot zones and disease progression in the northern US (Wyoming and Idaho) (Nakazawa et al., 2007).

These examples illustrate that more investigation is required to co-relate the complex interaction between environmental changes and intermittent reservoirs in order to validate the prediction of plague transmission.

6.3.5 Newer Modalities: Prediction Methods

In recent years, clinical reports of pneumonic plague have been documented in Madagascar. Taking this into account, in an Infodemiological study using Google Trends (GT), the best regression model (1-day lag model) was generated for forecasting plague by correlating GT and epidemiological real-world statistics (relating incidence rate and spread pattern). This GT can provide significant data to track and monitor plague in real time at the earliest possible moment, before it is officially declared by the WHO (Bragazzi et al., 2019).

The application of artificial intelligence and machine learning approaches to the assessment of biological assays related to *Y. pestis* can provide us with better therapeutics and predictive measures, as suggested by Korotcov (Korotcov et al., 2017). A deep learning algorithm-based model can potentiate the image-driven data (spatial data) obtained from different geographical locations and helps in co-relating the patients' magnetic resonance imaging (MRI) diagnosis data (Winkler et al., 2021).

6.4 DENGUE

6.4.1 Introduction

Dengue, or dengue fever, is a viral disease caused by four different serotypes of dengue virus: DENV-1, DENV-2, DENV-3, and DENV-4. Dengue is a mosquito-borne single-stranded RNA virus of the Flaviviridae family that is transmitted (from mosquitoes to humans and vice versa) by female mosquitoes, primarily the species *Aedes aegypti* and *Aedes albopictus* (Murugesan et al., 2020; Messina et al., 2014). These mosquito vectors are also responsible for the transmission of chikungunya, yellow fever, and Zika viruses. Natural recovery against dengue confers life-long immunity but cross-reactivity shows partial recovery against other serotypes of the virus. Dengue can infect infants, young children, and adults. Infected people show mild to moderate flu-like symptoms, depending upon the immune system of the host (Messina et al., 2014; Hasan et al., 2016). If it is not managed well, death can happen. Almost half the world's population has faced epidemic and pandemic dengue. Each year, 400 million people are infected by dengue, and 40,000 deaths are reported in the WHO 2021 report. The worldwide risk of dengue depends upon changes in climatic parameters and environmental factors (Wang et al., 2020).

6.4.2 Dengue Vector Ecology and Distribution

It is well known that environmental conditions influence the survival and multiplication of the dengue vectors. *Aedes* mosquitoes such as *Aedes aegypti* and *Aedes albopictus* are primary vectors for the spread of disease. *Aedes* mosquitoes are generally distributed in the tropical and temperate areas of Africa, Asia, America, Australia, the South Pacific, and some parts of the Middle East. *Ae. aegypti* prefers to grow in tropical and dry areas, whereas *Ae. albopictus* has adapted to grow in tropical to temperate regions (Hawley et al., 1988). The life cycle of *Aedes* is completely dependent on the natural and man-made environment. The larvae breed in natural and artificial habitats such as standing water deposited in tree holes, discarded plastic containers, flower pots, open water tanks, ant traps, and discarded vehicle tyres around human residences (Higa et al., 2011).

In general, *Aedes aegypti* shows multiplication in the domestic environment of the urban area, which indicates their growth adaptation to the urban area. However, *Aedes albopictus* distribution is associated with vegetation throughout rural and urban areas (Tsuda et al., 2006).

6.4.3 Impact of Climatic Factors on Dengue

The growth kinetics of dengue fever significantly depends upon climatic factors such as temperature, rainfall, and relative humidity. It has been noted that the rainy season and post-monsoon time are the most favourable time for mosquito multiplication and transmission of the dengue virus.

Many Asian country researchers have mentioned that temperature is a major climatic factor that is strongly associated with dengue fever incidence. The most favourable temperature range for the multiplication of the dengue virus (*Aedes aegypti*) was found to be 24–31 °C (Tuladhar et al., 2019).

> Apart from temperature, rainfall and sunshine are both negatively associated with dengue fever incidence. Heavy rainfall disrupts the breeding cycle of mosquitoes and washes their eggs and larvae from breeding sites. Warmer temperature promotes mosquito growth up to a certain limit, but longer hours of sunshine (heat) may not promote mosquito density. Higher temperature generates more heat, which can affect larval growth (Lai et al., 2018).

It has been reported that the mosquitoes' life span is reduced at humidity lower than 60%, disrupting the vector efficiency. However, the life span of mosquitoes increased in the presence of 80% humidity at optimal temperature, leading to an increase in the transmission rate of dengue and the occurrence of dengue fever (Monintja et al., 2021).

An autoregressive model, ARMAX, predicts the relationship between dengue incidence and climatic factors. On the other hand, the optimal model represents that wind speed, humidity, and rainfall are negatively associated with dengue incidence (Xavier et al., 2021).

6.4.4 Prevention and Treatment

At present, there are no allopathic medicines available for the cure of dengue. Anti-inflammatory medicines such as acetaminophen are used when dengue fever has been confirmed. A medicine such as aspirin should be avoided, as it can enhance bleeding during infection. Reports suggested that plenty of fluids and rest should be taken during infection. The best way to prevent dengue fever is to protect oneself from the bite of an infected mosquito and destroy water logging around the home.

In 2019, a vaccine against the dengue virus, Dengvaxia (CYD-TDV), was approved by the Food and Drug Administration (FDA). Dengvaxia is a recombinant tetravalent vaccine against the dengue infection, developed by Sanofi Pasteur. Dengvaxia (CYD-TDV) can be taken from below the age of 9 to 45 years old (WHO, 2018) when dengue infection is confirmed in the patient (WHO, Vaccines and immunization: Dengue, 2018).

Recently, a genetically modified symbiotic *Wolbachia* bacterium has been introduced, which can affect the cellular and metabolic mechanism of the *Aedes* mosquito vector. This bacterium alters the sexual cycle of the vector, which is responsible for the decreasing population of mosquitoes (Rather et al., 2017).

An herbaceous medicinal plant called papaya (*Carica papaya* L.) has been used as a traditional medicine for the cure of dengue infection in India. It has been reported in the literature that papaya seeds are toxic to *Aedes aegypti*, and papaya leaves showed haemolytic-inhibitory effects against dengue. Papaya can promote platelet counts and increase the production of thrombocytes (Manohar, 2013).

6.5 ENCEPHALITIS

6.5.1 Background

Encephalitis is a type of brain parenchymal inflammation causing neurological dysfunctions and other problems such as headache, fever, loss of consciousness, epileptic seizures, problems with speech or hearing, and behavioural changes (Costa et al., 2020; Kennedy, 2004). A number of factors can cause encephalitis, but the most common cause is viral infection or autoimmunity. Herpes simplex virus, Epstein–Barr virus, enteroviruses, mosquito-borne viruses, tick-borne viruses, rabies virus, measles (rubeola), mumps, German measles (rubella) viruses, and other viruses are mainly responsible for causing viral encephalitis. Apart from viral infection, several other neurological disorders may cause encephalitis without brain tissue inflammation (Tyler, 2018). As per the literature, up to the age of 2, approximately 16 per 100,000 children are affected annually. Up to the age of 15, 1/100,000 children are affected yearly. Polymerase chain reaction (PCR) and brain imaging techniques such as computed tomography,

MRI, and electroencephalography (EEG) are major diagnostic tools for the confirmation of disease. The frequency of encephalitis may also be affected by the viral mutation rate, the geographical location, and the patient's immunological status (Saxena et al., 2009).

Japanese encephalitis (JE) is the most common viral encephalitis in Asia, caused by the JE virus, which mainly affects brain parenchyma and causes symptoms like fever, headache, and epileptic seizures (Xu Chongxiao et al., 2022). It is a mosquito-borne disease transmitted by the *Culex* mosquito (*Culex tritaeniorhynchus*) and belongs to the same Flavivirus family as dengue, yellow fever, and West Nile viruses. JE has affected 24 countries in Southeast Asia and the Western Pacific Rim. It has been noted that 30% of Japanese encephalitis virus (JEV)-affected patients died in hospital. Approximately 68,000 clinical cases of JE have been reported annually worldwide (Kulkarni et al., 2018).

6.5.2 Ecological Parameters and Climatic Factors Associated with Encephalitis Transmission

In the last 30 years, the world has experienced the outbreak and emergence of many infectious diseases, either zoonotic or vector-borne (Waits Audrey et al., 2018). Zoonotic and vector-borne diseases are indirectly affected by environmental factors, especially temperature, precipitation, and humidity. The principal mechanisms by which a warm climate modulates the host–pathogen interaction include host population, vector adaptability, increment in pathogen survival, and virus mutation rate (Burek et al., 2008). It has been reported that relatively minor temperature change can create a new environmental niche for the habitats, which can introduce a new host–pathogen relationship and increase the vector range (Dudley et al., 2015).

The tick-borne diseases are the most common infectious diseases allied with climatic factors. As per reports, temperature and precipitation significantly enhance the life cycle and distribution of ticks, indirectly affecting the transmission of tick-borne encephalitis in Europe and Russia (Semenza Jan et al., 2009). In contrast to climatic factors, Finland-based researchers found that animal density could be positively associated with the incidence of tick-borne encephalitis. They selected five animals (moose, roe-deer, white-tailed deer, mountain hare, and red fox) in the game management area of Finland from 2007 to 2017. Of these five animals, the white-tailed deer was positively associated with encephalitis disease transmission; however, the others were not affected by disease burden (Dub et al., 2020).

A study from Asian countries (China, Taiwan, Vietnam, Nepal, and India) showed that climatic factors such as temperature, rainfall, relative humidity, and solar radiation significantly affect JE cases (Kumar Pant et al., 2017). These factors influence JE disease by larval development in a short time and mosquito population density (Murty et al., 2010). It has been reported that in the presence of warm weather, the replication rate and transmission of the virus increase (Kilpatrick et al., 2008).

6.5.3 Vaccination and Therapeutic Approach to Encephalitis

At present, there is no specific medicine available for providing a 100% cure for encephalitis. However, precautions and proper care could be beneficial and help in recovery from the JE virus infection. Doctors advise that the care room should be properly aerated and ventilated around the patient during the whole day and maintained appropriately. Plenty of water and electrolytes should be taken on a timely basis to stay hydrated and maintain acid–base balance in the body. In the case of fever, suitable antipyretics and cooling systems should be used. Epileptic seizures are effectively managed by anti-convulsion medicines such as phenytoin and valproate. If the intracranial pressure rises, then diuretics such as mannitol infusion (0.25 to 1.0 mg/kg every 4 to 6 hours) or intravenous furosemide may be given (Kumar, 2020).

Vaccine is an alternative and economical approach to the control of viral encephalitis. The lack of a mass vaccination programme resulted in people facing severe encephalitis in the epidemic areas of Asian countries. Initially, a vaccine for encephalitis was developed in mouse brain cells. In 1980, a China-based virologist developed a live attenuated SA 14-14-2 JE vaccine (LAJEV), which is grown in the primary kidney cells of hamsters. LAJEV has been used in several Asian countries, including India (Hombach et al., 2005).

At present, about 15 JE vaccines have been developed and commercialised in Asia. They fall into four categories: (1) live attenuated vaccines (i.e., CD-LAJEV); (2) live recombinant (chimeric) vaccines (i.e., JE-CV); (3) Vero cell-derived inactivated vaccines; and (4) mouse brain-derived inactivated vaccines (Vannice et al., 2021; Borah et al., 2013).

6.6 CONCLUSION AND REMARKS

Zoonotic diseases and components of climate at both micro and macro level are interrelated. Several studies have reported that zoonotic plague infections have links with weather variations. The potential factors, elements, and parameters that may possibly be related to spatial changes or long-term climate changes have been discussed.

It has been noted that advanced scales are needed for more accurate forecasting of zoonotic diseases. Satellite-driven sensing, geo-sensing techniques, etc. predict more real-time data on large scales. The intrinsic dynamics of zoonotic diseases with respect to vectors and primary/secondary hosts need to be related to meteorological parameters for the earliest prophylaxis. The primary measures implemented in the surveillance and prevention of zoonoses include understanding the natural cycles and behaviour of fleas, rodents, and mites, and implementing environmental management programmes. Long-term surveillance of the breeding activities of animal carriers will lead to a successful foundation to control zoonosis outbreaks. Scientific forecasting will be of utmost importance for health policymakers to focus on developing the health sector in underprivileged countries and reducing the zoonotic infections associated with weather variation.

These scientific predictions are also helpful for the UN to facilitate dealing with global warming and other serious climatic shifts.

REFERENCES

Ari, Tamara Ben, Alexander Gershunov, Rouyer Tristan, Bernard Cazelles, Kenneth Gage, and Nils C. Stenseth. "Interannual variability of human plague occurrence in the Western United States explained by tropical and North Pacific Ocean climate variability." *The American Journal of Tropical Medicine and Hygiene* 83, no. 3 (2010): 624.

Bartlow, Andrew W., Carrie Manore, Chonggang Xu, Kimberly A. Kaufeld, Sara Del Valle, Amanda Ziemann, Geoffrey Fairchild, and Jeanne M. Fair. "Forecasting zoonotic infectious disease response to climate change: Mosquito vectors and a changing environment." *Veterinary Sciences* 6, no. 2 (2019): 40.

Borah, Jani, Prafulla Dutta, Siraj A. Khan, and Jagadish Mahanta. "Association of weather and anthropogenic factors for transmission of Japanese encephalitis in an endemic area of India." *EcoHealth* 10, no. 2 (2013): 129–136.

Bragazzi, Nicola Luigi, and Naim Mahroum. "Google trends predicts present and future plague cases during the plague outbreak in Madagascar: Infodemiological study." *JMIR Public Health and Surveillance* 5, no. 1 (2019): e13142.

Burek, Kathy A., F. M. Gulland, T. M. O'Hara. "Effects of climate change on Arctic marine mammal health."*Ecological Applications* 18, no. sp2 (2008): S126–S134.

Caminade, Cyril, Sari Kovats, Joacim Rocklov, Adrian M. Tompkins, Andrew P. Morse, Felipe J. Colón-González, Hans Stenlund, Pim Martens, and Simon J. Lloyd. "Impact of climate change on global malaria distribution." *Proceedings of the National Academy of Sciences* 111, no. 9 (2014): 3286–3291.

Casimiro, Elsa, Jose Calheiros, Filipe Duarte Santos, and Sari Kovats. "National assessment of human health effects of climate change in Portugal: Approach and key findings." *Environmental Health Perspectives* 114, no. 12 (2006): 1950–1956.

"Cleveland clinic: Bubonic plague (black death): What is it, symptoms, treatment." (2021). Accessed: December 12, 2022. https://my.clevelandclinic.org/health/diseases/21590-bubonic-plague

Corder, Rodrigo M., Gilberto A. Paula, Anaclara Pincelli, and Marcelo U. Ferreira. "Statistical modeling of surveillance data to identify correlates of urban malaria risk: A population-based study in the Amazon Basin." *Plos One* 14, no. 8 (2019): e0220980.

Costa, Bruna Klein da, and Douglas Kazutoshi Sato. "Viral encephalitis: A practical review on diagnostic approach and treatment." *Jornal de Pediatria* 96 (2020): 12–19.

De Giusti, Maria, Domenico Barbato, Lorenza Lia, Vittoria Colamesta, Anna Maria Lombardi, Domenico Cacchio, Paolo Villari, and Giuseppe La Torre. "Collaboration between human and veterinary medicine as a tool to solve public health problems." *The Lancet Planetary Health* 3, no. 2 (2019): e64–e65.

Demeure, Christian E., Olivier Dussurget, Guillem Mas Fiol, Anne-Sophie Le Guern, Cyril Savin, and Javier Pizarro-Cerdá. "Yersinia pestis and plague: An updated view on evolution, virulence determinants, immune subversion, vaccination, and diagnostics." *Genes and Immunity* 20, no. 5 (2019): 357–370.

Dub, Timothee, Jukka Ollgren, Sari Huusko, Ruut Uusitalo, Mika Siljander, Olli Vapalahti, and Jussi Sane. "Game animal density, climate, and tick-borne encephalitis in Finland, 2007–2017." *Emerging Infectious Diseases* 26, no. 12 (2020): 2899.

Dudley, Joseph P., Eric P. Hoberg, Emily J. Jenkins, and Alan J. Parkinson. "Climate change in the North American Arctic: A one health perspective." *EcoHealth* 12, no. 4 (2015): 713–725.

Eisen, Lars, and Rebecca J. Eisen. "Using geographic information systems and decision support systems for the prediction, prevention, and control of vector-borne diseases." *Annual Review of Entomology* 56 (2011): 41–61.

Eisen, Rebecca J., and Kenneth L. Gage. "Adaptive strategies of Yersinia pestis to persist during inter-epizootic and epizootic periods." *Veterinary Research* 40, no. 2 (2009): 1.

Fauci, Anthony S., and David M. Morens. "The perpetual challenge of infectious diseases." *New England Journal of Medicine* 366, no. 5 (2012): 454–461.

Gage, Kenneth L., Thomas R. Burkot, Rebecca J. Eisen, and Edward B. Hayes. "Climate and vectorborne diseases." *American Journal of Preventive Medicine* 35, no. 5 (2008): 436–450.

Gneiting, Tilmann, and Adrian E. Raftery. "Atmospheric science. Weather forecasting with ensemble methods." *Science* 310, no. 5746 (2005): 248–249.

Hasan, Shamimul, Sami Faisal Jamdar, Munther Alalowi, and Al Beaiji Sadun Mohammad Al Ageel. "Dengue virus: A global human threat: Review of literature." *Journal of International Society of Preventive and Community Dentistry* 6, no. 1 (2016): 1.

Hawley, William A. "The biology of Aedes albopictus." *Journal of the American Mosquito Control Association. Supplement* 1 (1988): 1–39.

Health, Human, and National Research Council (US) Committee on Climate, Ecosystems, Infectious Diseases, and Human Health. "*Under the Weather: Climate, Ecosystems, and Infectious Disease.*" Washington (DC): National Academies Press (US), 2001.

Higa, Yukiko. "Dengue vectors and their spatial distribution." *Tropical Medicine and Health* 39, no. 4 (2011): S17–S27.

Holt, Ashley Christine. *Spatial and Temporal Dynamics of Plague in the United States: Historical, Recent, and Future Geographies.* Berkeley: University of California, 2009.

Hombach, Joachim, Tom Solomon, Ichiro Kurane, Julie Jacobson, and David Wood. "Report on a WHO consultation on immunological endpoints for evaluation of new Japanese encephalitis vaccines, WHO, Geneva, 2–3 September 2004." *Vaccine* 23, no. 45 (2005): 5205–5211.

Huber, Irene, Katerina Potapova, Elena Ammosova, Wolfgang Beyer, Sergey Blagodatskiy, Roman Desyatkin, Ludwig E. Hoelzle et al. "Symposium report: Emerging threats for human health–impact of socioeconomic and climate change on zoonotic diseases in the Republic of Sakha (Yakutia), Russia." *International Journal of Circumpolar Health* 79, no. 1 (2020): 1715698.

Joint, F. A. O., and World Health Organization. "*Joint WHO/FAO Expert Committee on Zoonoses [Meeting Held in Stockholm from 11 to 16 August 1958]: Second Report*". World Health Organization, (1959). Accessed: December 12, 2022. https://apps.who.int/iris/handle/10665/40435

Keiser, Jennifer, Marcia Caldas De Castro, Michael F. Maltese, Robert Bos, Marcel Tanner, Burton H. Singer, and Jurg Utzinger. "Effect of irrigation and large dams on the burden of malaria on a global and regional scale." *The American Journal of Tropical Medicine and Hygiene* 72, no. 4 (2005): 392–406.

Kennedy, P. G. E. "Viral encephalitis: Causes, differential diagnosis, and management." *Journal of Neurology, Neurosurgery, and Psychiatry* 75, no. Suppl 1 (2004): i10–i15.

Kilpatrick, A. Marm, Mark A. Meola, Robin M. Moudy, and Laura D. Kramer. "Temperature, viral genetics, and the transmission of West Nile virus by Culex pipiens mosquitoes." *Plos Pathogens* 4, no. 6 (2008): e1000092.

Korotcov, Alexandru, Valery Tkachenko, Daniel P. Russo, and Sean Ekins. "Comparison of deep learning with multiple machine learning methods and metrics using diverse drug discovery data sets." *Molecular Pharmaceutics* 14, no. 12 (2017): 4462–4475.

Krasnov, B. R., N. V. Burdelova, G. I. Shenbrot, and I. S. Khokhlova. "Annual cycles of four flea species in the central Negev Desert." *Medical and Veterinary Entomology* 16, no. 3 (2002): 266–276.

Krasnov, B. R., I. S. Khokhlova, L. J. Fielden, and N. V. Burdelova. "Development rates of two Xenopsylla flea species in relation to air temperature and humidity." *Medical and Veterinary Entomology* 15, no. 3 (2001): 249–258.

Kulkarni, Reshma, Gajanan N. Sapkal, Himanshu Kaushal, and Devendra T. Mourya. "M8: Japanese encephalitis: A brief review on Indian perspectives." *The Open Virology Journal* 12 (2018): 121–130.

Kumar, Rashmi. "Understanding and managing acute encephalitis." *F1000Research* 9 (2020): 60.

Lai, Yi-Horng. "The climatic factors affecting dengue fever outbreaks in southern Taiwan: An application of symbolic data analysis." *BioMedical Engineering Online* 17, no. 2 (2018): 1–14.

Leal Filho, Walter, Linda Ternova, Sanika Arun Parasnis, Marina Kovaleva, and Gustavo J. Nagy. "Climate change and zoonoses: A review of concepts, definitions, and bibliometrics." *International Journal of Environmental Research and Public Health* 19, no. 2 (2022): 893.

Lindsay, Steven W., David G. Hole, Robert A. Hutchinson, Shane A. Richards, and Stephen G. Willis. "Assessing the future threat from vivax malaria in the United Kingdom using two markedly different modelling approaches." *Malaria Journal* 9, no. 1 (2010): 1–8.

Magouras, Ioannis, Victoria J. Brookes, Ferran Jori, Angela Martin, Dirk Udo Pfeiffer, and Salome Dürr. "Emerging zoonotic diseases: Should we rethink the animal–human interface?" *Frontiers in Veterinary Science* 7 (2020): 582743.

Manohar, P. Ram. "Papaya, dengue fever and Ayurveda." *Ancient Science of Life* 32, no. 3 (2013): 131.

Martinez, Micaela Elvira. "The calendar of epidemics: Seasonal cycles of infectious diseases." *PLOS Pathogens* 14, no. 11 (2018): e1007327.

Messina, Jane P., Oliver J. Brady, Thomas W. Scott, Chenting Zou, David M. Pigott, Kirsten A. Duda, Samir Bhatt et al. "Global spread of dengue virus types: Mapping the 70 year history." *Trends in Microbiology* 22, no. 3 (2014): 138–146.

Monintja, Tyrsa C. N., A. Arsunan Arsin, Ridwan Amiruddin, and Muhammad Syafar. "Analysis of temperature and humidity on dengue hemorrhagic fever in Manado Municipality." *Gaceta Sanitaria* 35 (2021): S330–S333.

Murty, U., M. Suryanarayana, Srinivasa Rao, and N. Arunachalam. "The effects of climatic factors on the distribution and abundance of Japanese encephalitis vectors in Kurnool district of Andhra Pradesh, India." *Journal of Vector Borne Diseases* 47, no. 1 (2010): 26.

Murugesan, Amudhan, and Mythreyee Manoharan. Chapter 16-"Dengue virus." In Edited by Moulay Mustapha Ennaji *Emerging and Reemerging Viral Pathogens*, 281–359. London, Uk: Academic Press and Elsevier, 2020.

Nakazawa, Yoshinori, Richard Williams, A. Townsend Peterson, Paul Mead, Erin Staples, and Kenneth L. Gage. "Climate change effects on plague and tularemia in the United States." *Vector Borne and Zoonotic Diseases* 7, no. 4 (2007): 529–540.

Oliveria, B., A. P. de Moura, and L. M. Cunha. *Climate Change and Health Improving Resilience and Reducing Risks*, 117–132, 2016.

Pant, Dhan Kumar, Tenzin Tenzin, R. Chand, B. Kumar Sharma, and P. Raj Bist. "Spatio-temporal epidemiology of Japanese encephalitis in Nepal, 2007–2015." *Plos One* 12, no. 7 (2017): e0180591.

Parham, Paul Edward, and Edwin Michael. "Modeling the effects of weather and climate change on malaria transmission." *Environmental Health Perspectives* 118, no. 5 (2010): 620–626.

Parmenter, Robert R., Ekta Pratap Yadav, Cheryl A. Parmenter, Paul Ettestad, and Kenneth L. Gage. "Incidence of plague associated with increased winter-spring precipitation in New Mexico." *The American Journal of Tropical Medicine and Hygiene* 61, no. 5 (1999): 814–821.

Patz, Jonathan A., Diarmid Campbell-Lendrum, Tracey Holloway, and Jonathan A. Foley. "Impact of regional climate change on human health." *Nature* 438, no. 7066 (2005): 310–317.

"Plague - Annual epidemiological report for 2019." *European Centre for Disease Prevention and Control.* January 20, 2021.

Rather, Irfan A., Hilal A. Parray, Jameel B. Lone, Woon K. Paek, Jeongheui Lim, Vivek K. Bajpai, and Yong-Ha Park. "Prevention and control strategies to counter dengue virus infection." *Frontiers in Cellular and Infection Microbiology* 7 (2017): 336.

"RTS,S/AS01. "RTS,S - PATH's malaria vaccine initiative." (2019). Accessed: December 13, 2022. https://www.malariavaccine.org/malaria-and-vaccines/rtss.

Rupasinghe, Ruwini, Bruno B. Chomel, and Beatriz Martínez-López. "Climate change and zoonoses: A review of the current status, knowledge gaps, and future trends." *Acta Tropica* 226 (2022): 106225.

Saxena, V., K. M. Virendra, and N. D. Tapan. "Evaluation of reverse-transcriptase PCR as a diagnostic tool to confirm Japanese encephalitis virus infection." *Transactions of the Royal Society of Tropical Medicine and Hygiene* 103, no. 4 (2009): 403–406.

Schaechter, M., ed. *Eukaryotic Microbes*, 654–654. Amsterdam: Academic Press and Elsevier, 2012.

Semenza, Jan C., and Bettina Menne. "Climate change and infectious diseases in Europe." *The Lancet Infectious Diseases* 9, no. 6 (2009): 365–375.

Skea, Jim, Priyadarshi Shukla, Alaa Al. Khourdajie, and David McCollum. "Intergovernmental panel on climate change: Transparency and integrated assessment modeling." *Wiley Interdisciplinary Reviews: Climate Change* 12, no. 5 (2021): e727.

Smith, M. W., T. Willis, L. Alfieri, W. H. M. James, M. A. Trigg, D. Yamazaki, A. J. Hardy et al. "Incorporating hydrology into climate suitability models changes projections of malaria transmission in Africa." *Nature Communications* 11, no. 1 (2020): 1–9.

Stenseth, Nils Chr., Noelle I. Samia, Hildegunn Viljugrein, Kyrre Linné Kausrud, Mike Begon, Stephen Davis, Herwig Leirs et al. "Plague dynamics are driven by climate variation." *Proceedings of the National Academy of Sciences of the United States of America* 103, no. 35 (2006): 13110–13115.

Taylor, L. H., M. L. Sophia, and E. J. W. Mark. "Risk factors for human disease emergence." *Philosophical Transactions of the Royal Society of London. Series B: Biological Sciences* 356, no. 1411 (2001): 983–989.

Trottier, Helen, and Susan J. Elliott. "World Health Organization recommends first malaria vaccine." *Canadian Journal of Public Health* 112, no. 6 (2021): 967–969.

Tsuda, Yoshio, Wannapa Suwonkerd, Srisucha Chawprom, Somsak Prajakwong, and Masahiro Takagi. "Different spatial distribution of Aedes aegypti and Aedes albopictus along an urban–rural gradient and the relating environmental factors examined in three villages in northern Thailand." *Journal of the American Mosquito Control Association* 22, no. 2 (2006): 222–228.

Tuladhar, Reshma, Anjana Singh, Ajit Varma, and Devendra Kumar Choudhary. Climatic factors influencing dengue incidence in an epidemic area of Nepal." *BMC Research Notes* 12, no. 1 (2019): 1–7.

Tyler, Kenneth L. "Acute viral encephalitis." *New England Journal of Medicine* 379, no. 6 (2018): 557–566.

Vannice, Kirsten S., Susan L. Hills, Lauren M. Schwartz, Alan D. Barrett, James Heffelfinger, Joachim Hombach, G. William Letson, Tom Solomon, and Anthony A. Marfin. "The future of Japanese encephalitis vaccination: Expert recommendations for achieving and maintaining optimal JE control." *NPJ Vaccines* 6 (2021): 1–9.

Waits, Audrey, Anastasia Emelyanova, Antti Oksanen, Khaled Abass, and Arja Rautio. "Human infectious diseases and the changing climate in the Arctic." *Environment International* 121, no. 1 (2018): 703–713.

Wang, Wen-Hung, Aspiro Nayim Urbina, Max R. Chang, Wanchai Assavalapsakul, Po-Liang Lu, Yen-Hsu Chen, and Sheng-Fan Wang. "Dengue hemorrhagic fever–a systemic literature review of current perspectives on pathogenesis, prevention and control." *Journal of Microbiology, Immunology, and Infection* 53, no. 6 (2020): 963–978.

WHO. "Plague." (2022). Accessed: December 11, 2022. https https://www.who.int/news-room/fact-sheets/detail/plague

Winkler, David A. "Use of artificial intelligence and machine learning for discovery of drugs for neglected tropical diseases." *Frontiers in Chemistry* 9 (2021): 614073.

World Health Organization. "*Evaluation of Genetically Modified Mosquitoes for the Control of Vector-Borne Diseases: Position Statement*". (2020). Accessed: December 12, 2022. https://www.who.int/publications/i/item/9789240013155

World Health Organization. "*Vaccines and Immunization: Dengue*". (2018). Accessed: December 12, 2022. https://www.who.int/news-room/questions-and-answers/item/dengue-vaccines

Xavier, Leandro Layter, Nildimar Alves Honório, José Francisco Moreira Pessanha, and Paulo César Peiter. "Analysis of climate factors and dengue incidence in the metropolitan region of Rio de Janeiro, Brazil." *Plos One* 16, no. 5 (2021): e0251403.

Xu, Chongxiao, Weijia Zhang, Yuefeng Pan, Guowei Wang, Qikai Yin, Shihong Fu, Fan Li et al. "A bibliometric analysis of global research on Japanese encephalitis from 1934 to 2020." *Frontiers in Cellular and Infection Microbiology* 12 (2022): 8.

[illegible] Varma, and Devendra Kumar Chaudhary. "Climate [illegible]" [illegible]

[illegible] *New England Journal of Medicine* [illegible]

[illegible] Anna G. [illegible] Lu [illegible] Solomon [illegible] "The [illegible]" [illegible]

W[illegible] Khaled Abu [illegible] Ali [illegible] "[illegible] disease [illegible]" [illegible] 2019 [illegible]

Wang, Wei [illegible] [illegible] [illegible] Wang. "[illegible]" [illegible]

WHO [illegible] (2020). [illegible] https://[illegible]

[illegible] "[illegible]" [illegible]

[illegible] December [illegible] [illegible]

[illegible] Accessed December [illegible] 20[illegible]

[illegible] Layer [illegible]

Xu [illegible] Yuebo [illegible] [illegible]

7 Environmental Dimensions of Zika Virus Triggered Outbreak and Its Association with Neurological Complications Like Guillain–Barré Syndrome and Microcephaly

Ishfaq Ahmad Ahanger and Shah Ubaid-ullah

CONTENTS

7.1 Introduction 100
7.2 Environmental Dimension of Zika Virus Disease Outbreaks 101
7.2.1 Structural Features of Zika Virus Proteins 103
7.2.2 Management, Prevention, and Control 105
7.2.3 Associations of Zika Virus with Neurological Complications 105
7.2.3.1 Guillain–Barré Syndrome (GBS) 107
7.2.3.2 Microcephaly 109
7.2.3.3 Inflammation of Schwann Cells by Zika Virus 110
7.3 Concluding Remarks 110
Conflict of Interest 111
Acknowledgments 111
References 111

DOI: 10.1201/9781003288732-7

7.1 INTRODUCTION

Zika virus (ZIKV) is a mosquito-borne virus belonging to the *Flaviviridae* family, responsible for causing illness referred to as Zika virus disease or Zika fever (Wang et al., 2016). It is spread by the *Aedes* mosquito, which is also responsible for spreading the dengue and chikungunya viruses (Cardoso et al., 2015). Symptoms of the Zika virus disease may be absent, ambiguous, or mild; fever, rashes, joint discomfort, conjunctivitis or red eyes, muscular pain, headache, pain behind the eyes, and vomiting are some of the initial symptoms, which can persist for up to 1 week (Meaney-Delman et al., 2016). Nevertheless, Zika infections can also be fatal, particularly if a woman acquires the infection during pregnancy (Rather et al., 2017), as ZIKV can pass from mother to fetus (trans-placental transmission) (Egloff et al., 2020). Alternative methods of infection, such as through blood transfusion or sexual contact, are also possible, although these are considerably less common (Viennet et al., 2020). In an unborn fetus, the infection can result in a brain abnormality described as microcephaly – a disease wherein the baby's head is much smaller than normal, usually because of aberrant brain development (Wen et al., 2017). It has been reported that in comparison with previous years, there has been a tenfold rise in babies with microcephaly as a result of the latest pandemic in Brazil in October 2015 (Brady et al., 2019). Moreover, human beings have also developed Guillain–Barré syndrome (GBS) after being infected with the Zika virus (Carod-Artal, 2018). GBS is a neurological complication in which the immune system attacks the central nervous system, causing muscular rigidity (Oehler et al., 2014). This disease is characterised by unspecified symptoms; tingling in the feet or hands, or maybe even pain (particularly in infants) in the legs or back, are common at the onset. Children may also experience trouble walking and may be unwilling to walk. These feelings usually fade away before more serious, long-term problems develop (Krauer et al., 2017).

There is presently no medication for Zika. To avoid dehydration, a person experiencing signs must relax and maximise fluid intake. To treat discomfort and fever, over-the-counter pain relievers are a good choice (Mumtaz et al., 2016). Because of the risk of bleeding, the Centers for Disease Control (CDC) recommends avoiding aspirin or other non-steroidal anti-inflammatory medicines unless the diagnosis of dengue fever has been ruled out in individuals at risk. As per CDC guidelines, pregnant women who have been diagnosed with Zika should undergo fetal development and anatomy testing every 3 to 4 weeks (Agumadu and Ramphul, 2018). It is also suggested to consult a specialist in prenatal care, infectious illness, or maternal–fetal healthcare. Blood or urine testing could identify Zika disease, and many research labs conduct Zika testing, but that is not recommended if you are experiencing symptoms of Zika and have been to a place where the virus is currently spreading. Zika can be distinguished from other viral illnesses by means of ultrafast serologic polymerase chain reaction (PCR) tests performed 3–5 days after onset of symptoms (Faye et al., 2008). Other assays look for antibodies. Depending on the facility, screening can last anywhere from 2 to 4 weeks. Some persons may be clinically diagnosed during one global pandemic depending on individual indications and current history (Faye et al., 2008). A pregnant female transmits Zika to her fetus. Most birth abnormalities are caused by infection during pregnancy. Zika virus is also transmitted from an infected individual to his or her sex partners during intercourse. ZIKV infects the amniotic fluid and the embryonic central nervous system after crossing the placenta and has a major influence on neurodevelopment. Diseased brains are tiny, featuring larger ventricles and a weaker cortex, indicating a microcephalic phenotype (Ornelas et al., 2017). Yellow Fever Research Institute scientists originally isolated the virus in April 1947 from a rhesus macaque monkey kept in a cage in the forest of Uganda, near Lake Victoria. The finding of a serological investigation in Uganda, reported in 1952, was the first report to show that Zika could infect humans. Because Zika infection in expectant mothers can typically cause congenital Zika syndrome in newborns, vaccination may protect from congenital Zika syndrome as a result of future outbreaks (Schwartz, 2017).

7.2 ENVIRONMENTAL DIMENSION OF ZIKA VIRUS DISEASE OUTBREAKS

The female *Aedes aegypti* mosquito is responsible for the transmission of Zika virus disease. The transmission occurs during the day, as *Aedes aegypti* is usually active during the daytime. The prevalence of the mosquito vectors that carry Zika could be used to analyse the possibility of community threat. Because of worldwide trade and travel, the most common Zika vector, *Aedes aegypti*, is spreading across the globe. *Aedes aegypti* has become widespread, encompassing sections of every hemisphere, including Antarctica, as well as North America and the European periphery (Kraemer et al., 2015). A Zika-carrying mosquito species has been identified in Washington. The genomic data from these vectors indicates that larvae have lived at least 4 years in the area. Mosquitoes are adjusting to survive in a northern environment, according to the scientists who carried out this investigation (Monaghan et al., 2016). Once transmitted, the Zika virus seems to be communicable by mosquitoes for about a week. When transferred by sperm, the virus is expected to be persistent for a greater duration, up to about 2 weeks following infection. According to one study, Zika transmission is impacted by variations in rainfall and temperature to a greater extent than dengue, and the chances are high that it will be restricted to tropical environments. Increased temperatures, on the other hand, could permit the infectious carrier to increase its area, thus enabling Zika to emerge (Carlson et al., 2016).

ZIKV data remained restricted to several geographical places in Africa and Asia before 2007, so the overall risk mapping was not really a focus. In 2013, the virus started spreading to other regions of Oceania, and in 2015, Brazil became the epicentre of a massive epidemic in Latin America. Reports depicted that there was a prominent connection between microcephaly and Guillain–Barré syndrome in the outbreak that occurred in the

Federated States of Micronesia, regions of Oceania, and Brazil. Popular concern regarding the sustained and growing prevalence of the virus caused the World Health Organization (WHO) to declare it a Public Health Emergency of International Concern. It has been reported that there are approximately 2.17 billion individuals living within the tropical and sub-tropical regions around the world that have adequate climatic conditions for the survival of this infection (Messina et al., 2016).

According to Peter Hotez, the *Aedes* mosquito has thrived due to 'environmental damage' in crucial places in Brazil and other nations. It also suggests that mosquitoes breed in areas such as rotting rubbish, dumped and submerged tyres, and standing water, and subsequently spread dangerous viruses (Mooney, 2016). Building dams is also said to be a vital factor that has contributed to the occurrence of Zika virus infection. Damming a huge body of water to utilise it for electricity or even to construct reservoirs is among the most environmentally damaging processes (Mooney, 2016). Most people have complained about the different ways in which these dams harm habitats; nevertheless, it is established now that dams alter aqueous habitats, which might promote vector-borne illness. The construction of dams is among the most important causes of the spread of schistosomiasis; for example, the dam on the Upper Volta aided in the vast spread of schistosomiasis in Ghana. Schistosomiasis, commonly termed snail fever (Chala and Torben, 2018), is triggered by parasitic flatworms known as schistosomes. Infection of the urinary system or intestines is possible as a result of this disease. Intestinal discomfort, diarrhoea, bloody stool, and blood in the urine are some of the symptoms. Long-term infection can lead to hepatic injury, nephrotic syndrome, impotence, and bladder cancer (Chala and Torben, 2018). Habitat destruction is once again a factor for malaria in Africa, where it is most deadly. Since deforested areas lack the cooling impact of forests, these regions are likely to be hotter, and this higher temperature might impair important aspects of the mosquito life cycle. It has been seen that female *Anopheles gambiae* mosquitoes have become lethal in Kenya due to massive deforested regions. Cutting or burning and looting trees has been linked to an increase in infectious diseases of humans (Mooney, 2016; Tunali et al., 2021). Deforestation can contribute to global warming. In addition, deforestation and increasing global temperatures may alter the suitable habitats of a wide variety of species, particularly disease-carrying insects. According to the WHO, in a humid environment, *Aedes aegypti* and all the diseases it carries are predicted to proliferate (Mooney, 2016). At extremely elevated temperatures, dengue mosquitoes multiply very rapidly and infect more routinely. According to a recent collaborative survey by US mosquito control scientists from numerous governmental bodies and Rutgers University, it is clear that *Aedes albopictus* has now spread over most of the US, and environmental degradation would accelerate its expansionist growth (Mooney, 2016; Wilke et al., 2019).

Thus, it can be concluded that there are marked consequences for the environment and ecosystem of various species, including mosquitoes, due to climate change (Asad and Carpenter, 2018). A rise in atmospheric temperature leads to global warming and fluctuating precipitation periods; humidity influences the endurance of eggs, and wind can alter the spatial dispersal of mosquitoes. These are some important determinants that have marked consequences for the environment and ecosystem of various species, including mosquitoes (Asad and Carpenter, 2018). All these factors depict the significant impact of climate change on the spread of viruses and are responsible for the upsurge in mosquito vector ranges, resulting in massive spread of Zika virus infection (Asad and Carpenter, 2018).

7.2.1 Structural Features of Zika Virus Proteins

The genome of Zika virus codes for at least ten proteins, three of which are structural (protein E, protein C, and protein prM) and seven of which are non-structural (NS1, NS2A, NS2B, NS3, NS4A, NS4B, and NS5) as shown in Figure 7.1. The flavivirus surface is primarily made up of protein E. This protein plays an important role in the recognition of host cell receptors, virus invasion, and viral assembly (Rather et al., 2017). It is indeed important to note that the virus–host cell endosomal membrane fusion is mediated via conformational changes in protein E caused by pH variations from extracellular to endosomal environments (Shi and Gao, 2017).

E protein plays a crucial role in the immunological response, as it is the primary target of neutralising antibodies. It is composed of three main domains: domain I (DI), domain II (DII), and domain III (DIII). As previously stated, protein E is the primary focus of the immune response towards flaviviruses, and

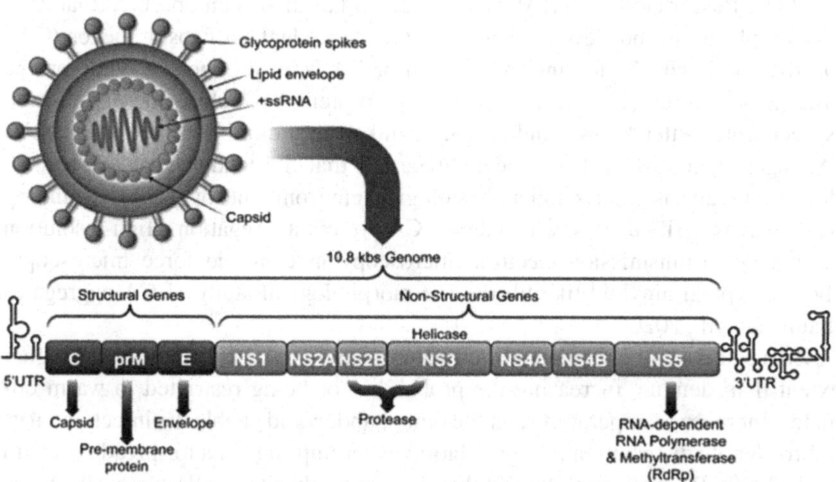

FIGURE 7.1 Diagrammatic representation of Zika virus genome and associated three structural proteins, (i) capsid (C), (ii) precursor of membrane (prM), and (iii) envelope (E), and seven non-structural proteins (NS1, NS2A, NS2B, NS3, NS4A, NS4B, and NS5). (From Rombi, F., et al., *Mol. Biol. Rep.*, 47, 3097, 2020.)

ZIKV is no exception (Kostyuchenko et al., 2016). As a result, portrayal of protein E's morphological and structural shifts, as well as its interactions with various antibodies, is required for the development of ZIKV vaccines or maybe even novel passive immunisation methods based on optimised antibodies or antibody fragments, such as the fragment antigen-binding (Fab) and the single-chain variable fragment, scFv (Beaver et al., 2018). The capsid (C) protein is a multifunctional protein that interacts with cellular proteins; modulates cellular metabolism, apoptosis, and the immune response; and attaches to viral RNA during nucleocapsid construction. Therefore, the major function of C protein is interaction with RNA, resulting in the formation of nucleocapsid. NS1 is a ~48-kDa protein that forms a part of replication complex organised with the transmembrane proteins. prM is responsible for maintenance, helping the folding of E protein (Valente and Moraes, 2019).

The vacuoles and mitochondria in cells tend to enlarge after 6 hours once the cell is infected with the Zika virus. When the enlargement becomes too extreme, the cells die, a process called paraptosis (Monel et al., 2017). Gene expression is considered an essential part of planned cell death. Interferon-induced transmembrane protein-3 (IFITM3) is a cell transmembrane protein that protects the cell against viral illness by preventing virus adherence. Whenever IFITM3 numbers are reduced, cells are more vulnerable to Zika infection (Gobillot et al., 2020). Once a cell is infected, the virus reorganises the endoplasmic reticulum, leading to the formation of enormous vacuoles and cell death. It has been found that Zika virus is involved in neurological complications such as Guillain–Barré syndrome and microcephaly. It is a well-established fact that generally, these neurological complications are coupled with protein misfolding and aggregation (Ahanger et al., 2021; Bashir et al., 2021;Ahanger, 2021). It has also been observed that Zika virus replication and development are both dependent on capsid anchor (CA). On the one hand, the folding mechanism of CA is as yet unclear, while on the other hand, the tendency to transmembrane protein misfolding and aggregation is becoming better known and has been linked to a number of proteinopathies (Ahanger et al., 2021). It has been suggested that the tendency of CA to produce aggregates is greater under physiological environments by using dye binding tests such as ThT kinetics, which depict CA protein aggregation. High-resolution microscopy (transmission electron microscopy and atomic force microscopy) showed typical amyloid-like fibrils in a morphological study of CA aggregates (Saumya et al., 2020).

Zika could well be regulated by climate variability and temperature to a higher extent than dengue, increasing the probability of being restricted to warm climates. Increased temperatures, on the other hand, could enable the infection virus to broaden its distribution in higher latitudes, prompting Zika to spread (Ferreira et al., 2020). Regardless of the fact that there are only a few full-length Zika virus sequences readily accessible, molecular studies are enough to reveal the pattern of viral evolution and mobility. The infection is thought to have started in East Africa and travelled to West Africa and ultimately to Asia, leading to different generations (Faye et al., 2014).

7.2.2 Management, Prevention, and Control

Medication for basic Zika virus infection is similar to that for other mosquito-borne flaviviruses. Because there is currently no Zika virus vaccine that has been licensed by the Food and Drug Administration (FDA), deterrence and management efforts are focused on minimising mosquito exposure, minimising sexual transmission, and managing the spread of the mosquito. Several experimental treatments are being tested, with preliminary human testing underway. No vaccines have been licensed for therapeutic application since about April 2019, even though a variety of vaccines are presently being tested in clinical trials (Abbink et al., 2018). A Zika virus vaccine's purpose should be to develop specific antibodies against the Zika virus in order to stop infection and serious illness. Trying to restrict complications like Guillain–Barré syndrome, which can occur due to Zika virus infection, is one of the issues in implementing a safe and reliable vaccine. Furthermore, because dengue virus and Zika virus are closely linked, the vaccination must reduce the risk of dengue virus infection. Phase I clinical studies are underway for a live attenuated vaccine wherein the virus has been biologically altered such that it cannot induce illness in people. This vaccine has been developed on the basis of Dengvaxia, a dengue vaccine that has been authorised for medical treatment. A redesigned mRNA vaccine incorporating the E and PrM proteins, developed in association with Moderna Therapeutics, is undertaking stage I and II clinical studies at the very same time (Taybeh, 2020).

Avoiding travel to regions where Zika virus propagation is underway, avoiding unsafe sexual relations with contacts who may be in danger of Zika virus infection, and using mosquito bug sprays, permethrin treatment for clothing, bed netting, frame curtains, and air-conditioning systems are all possibly good mitigation strategies that are aimed at minimising illness among expectant mothers. A pregnant woman must be subjected to blood examination and an ultrasound. The recommended strategy to diagnose Zika infection is to perform molecular amplification, i.e., reverse transcription (RT)-PCR, on blood serum, collected after 7 days following the onset of symptoms (Cao-Lormeau et al., 2014). Indications of the Zika virus have no particular therapy. Taking paracetamol and drinking plenty of fluids can help to alleviate discomfort. If you have been to a place where malaria is present as well as danger of Zika virus transmission, you should seek medical assistance (within 24 hours) and go for screening or diagnosis. Due to the obvious danger of bleeding in individuals suffering from dengue, aspirin as well as other non-steroidal anti-inflammatory drugs must be avoided unless dengue is ruled out (Županc and Petrovec, 2016).

7.2.3 Associations of Zika Virus with Neurological Complications

Zika virus outbreaks and congenital microcephaly appear to have geographical and historical correlations according to present epidemiological records (Županc and Petrovec, 2016). This is based on the fact that the virus is found in amniotic fluid or brain tissue of infected fetuses. To see if there is any link between

Zika virus infection and microcephaly, rigorous epidemiological investigations with specific criteria of microcephaly are being conducted (Županc and Petrovec, 2016). Zika virus infection causes cellular metabolic remodelling by inhibiting the mTOR pathway and activating p53 in neural stem cells, as depicted in Figure 7.2. Microcephaly is most commonly caused by improper brain growth. Microcephaly has no widely recognised classification (de Araújo et al., 2018). The Brazilian health authority (MoH) currently defines microcephaly as a head size just under two standard deviations below the average for sex and maternal age at birth (de Araújo et al., 2018).

The province of Paraba, in Northeast Brazil, has recorded almost 85% percent of the total occurrence of microcephaly since November 2015. It is unclear whether this represents an actual rise, a spike in serious conditions, or an upsurge in detection. In Colombia, where the Zika virus has been prevalent from October 2015, approximately 30,000 instances of Zika virus infection have been documented, with over 5,000 of them being in expectant mothers. There has been no evidence of related instances of microcephaly as yet (Basarab et al., 2016).

Brazil recorded 5,280 probable instances of microcephaly and/or central nervous system abnormality, involving 108 fatalities, between November 2015 and February 2016, and 1,345 of them were researched further: 837 of the 1,345

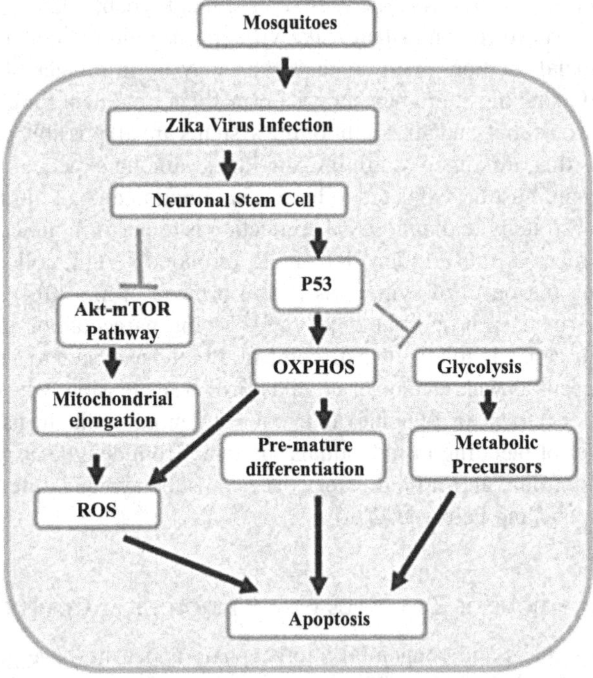

FIGURE 7.2 Zika virus infection causes cellular metabolic remodelling by inhibiting the mTOR pathway and activating P53 in neural stem cells.

people did not show microcephaly, 421 had radiological abnormalities such as cerebral calcium deposits that might indicate prenatal transmission, and 41 had verified Zika virus infection (Rodríguez-Barraquer et al., 2016).

7.2.3.1 Guillain–Barré Syndrome (GBS)

GBS is a neurological disorder in which the immune system targets the central nervous system, resulting in muscle stiffness (Van den Berg et al., 2014). Unresponsiveness, trembling, and aching, when in conjunction, are indeed the earliest signs of Guillain–Barré syndrome (Reyna-Villasmil et al., 2016). These are accompanied by leg and arm stiffness that hurts on both sides equally and becomes severe with the passage of time. The impairment usually takes anywhere from half a day to 2 weeks to reach its peak intensity, after which it remains stable. In around one out of every five patients, the stiffness persists for up to 4 weeks (Reyna-Villasmil et al., 2016).

Health professionals and virologists have struggled to validate the link between GBS and ZIKV infection due to the difficulty in showing ZIKV infection. The identification of Zika virus disease is dependent on the discovery of particular antibodies after the virus has disappeared from the blood. This method of verifying ZIKV disease has significant drawbacks in the setting of neurodevelopmental problems. In many instances, ZIKV is eliminated from blood by the time neurological symptoms appear (Cao-Lormeau et al., 2016; Parra et al., 2016). The muscles of the neckline might be involved, and in roughly half of those who have it, there is involvement of the cranial nerves that nourish the head and face, which results in muscle paralysis, chewing difficulty, and eye muscle pain. It is rare for the muscles that regulate the bladder and anus to be involved. Around one-third of persons suffering from GBS are still capable of walking. Gradually they may not be able to walk and this disability stays at a constant level before reaching equilibrium period. The equilibrium period might last anywhere from 2 to 6 months, although the most usual period is 7 days (Reyna-Villasmil, López-Sánchez, and Santos-Bolívar 2016).

Lumbar discomfort, uncomfortable sensations, muscle aches, and pain in the head and neck associated with stimulation of the brain tissue impact more than half of the affected population. It has been suggested that an attack by the immune system on peripheral nervous system neurons and their subsidiary components is responsible for nerve impairment in GBS (Nobuhiro and Hartung, 2012). Moreover, the brain and spine are encased in cerebrospinal fluid, and lumbar puncture, also known as spinal tap, is the evacuation of a tiny portion of this liquid with a syringe implanted between the lumbar vertebrae. GBS is defined by an increased protein content (typically higher than 0.55 g/L) and a low number of white blood cells per cubic millimetre of liquid (known as albumin-cytological dissociation) (Ropper, 1992). The foremost neurological illness linked to the Brazilian ZIKV epidemic was published in July 2015, after medical officials alerted the MoH to an increase in the number of GBS patients in the region of central northeastern Brazil. Following that, the WHO received notification regarding the upsurge in GBS cases in other South American nations. In October

2015, there were claims of a rise in the number of offspring born with microcephaly in the Brazilian state of Pernambuco, which was reported to the WHO.

In spite of mounting evidence of a link between ZIKV and GBS, the mechanisms underlying GBS development remain unknown. GBS is traditionally assumed to be immune facilitated, comprising cellular as well as humoral immune responses (Anaya et al., 2016). Molecular mimicry among some infections and the peripheral nervous system is one of the key proposed pathogenic pathways. Various reasons, particularly molecular mimicry, have been proposed as plausible pathogenic processes in the context of ZIKV-coupled GBS. Human proteins associated with myelination, axonal function, and neurodevelopment have been found to mimic ZIKV polyprotein (Anaya et al., 2016). Possible steps involved in the stimulation of TLR3 by Zika virus infection cause a metabolic imbalance of glycolysis. This ultimately results in massive amounts of reactive oxygen species (ROS) production when mitochondrial activity is inhibited, leading to neuronal cell malfunction and the formation of neurodegenerative disorders, including GBS, as shown in Figure 7.3.

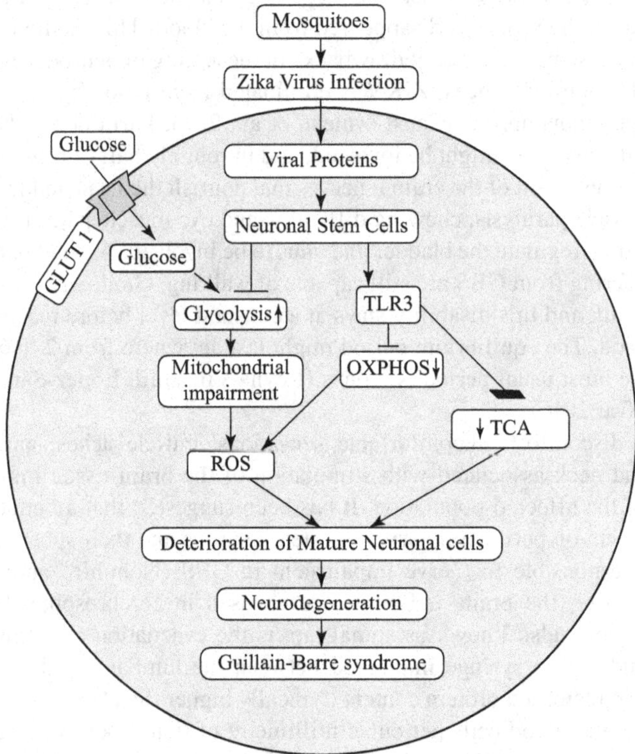

FIGURE 7.3 The stimulation of TLR3 by Zika virus infection causes a metabolic imbalance of glycolysis. Massive amounts of reactive oxygen species (ROS) are produced when mitochondrial activity is inhibited, leading to neuronal cell malfunction and the formation of neurodegenerative disorders, including Guillain–Barré syndrome.

7.2.3.2 Microcephaly

Microcephaly is a disorder in which a baby's head is significantly smaller than usual, generally due to abnormal neurodevelopment. In infants, there seem to be a range of indications that might appear (Faheem et al., 2015). Zika virus infection causes physiological disturbances in neural stem cells during the preliminary phase of differentiation, halting cellular proliferation and causing abrupt differentiation and death. At mature phases of neuronal cells, metabolic imbalances cause physiological malfunction and neurodegenerative disorders such as microcephaly, shown in Figure 7.4.

Congenital Zika syndrome is another name for this condition. Infants experiencing microcephaly will have either a regular or just a smaller head circumference when they are newborn. As a result, the head stops growing, whereas the face develops normally, resulting in a youngster with a tiny head, a receding skull, and a floppy, furrowed skull. Even as the child continues to grow, the shortness of the head becomes much more obvious, despite the fact that the whole physique is

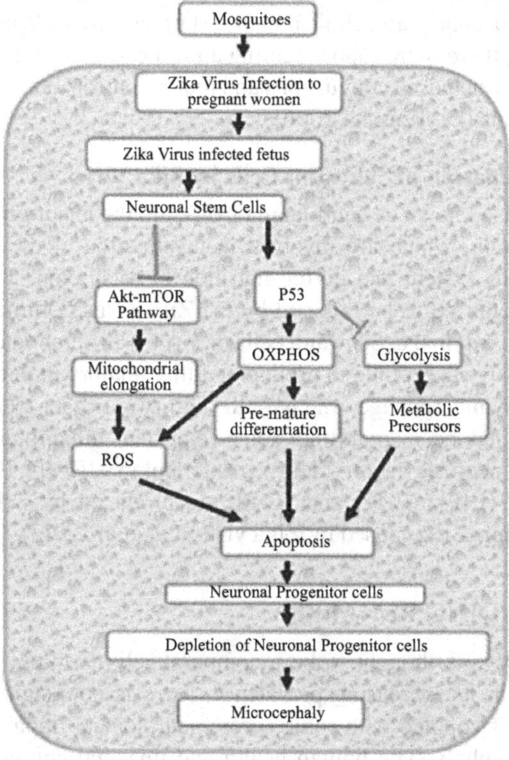

FIGURE 7.4 Zika virus infection causes physiological disturbances in neural stem cells during a preliminary phase of differentiation, halting cellular proliferation and causing abrupt differentiation and death. At mature phases of neuronal cells, metabolic imbalances cause physiological malfunction and neurodegenerative disorders such as microcephaly.

generally malnourished and undersized as well (Faheem et al., 2015). Although seriously hampered mental development is prevalent, motor coordination problems may well not manifest before older age. Neurobiological abnormalities and convulsions are common in these babies. Motor coordination and voice acquisition might well be disrupted (Ben-Zeev et al., 2003). Hyperactivity and mental retardation are both frequent, albeit the severity within each differs. Convulsions are also possible. The range of motor function is wide, extending from incompetence to severe quadriplegia in some (Ben-Zeev et al., 2003). During the epidemic in Brazil in 2015, the link between ZIKV and microcephaly abnormalities was initially recognised. The present published prevalence of 20 instances of microcephaly in every 10,000 live births is significantly higher than the projected average (Valentine et al., 2016). The increasing prevalence of microcephaly that corresponded to the ZIKV outbreak revealed a link between the virus and microcephaly. It has been observed that two expectant mothers in the northeast of Brazil were discovered to have abnormal outcomes of RT-PCR in the amniotic fluid of newborns with microcephaly, which is certainly adding to the concern (Valentine et al., 2016). Microcephaly has no established treatment. Since certain instances of microcephaly and clinical manifestations have been caused by amino acid deficiencies, therapy by supplementing amino acids has been found to ameliorate complaints including convulsions and motor control abnormalities in some of these individuals (De Koning, 2006).

7.2.3.3 Inflammation of Schwann Cells by Zika Virus

Schwann cells, also known as neurolemmocytes, are the major glia of the peripheral nervous system, which are involved in myelination of the neurons of the peripheral nervous system and giving nutrition to each axon. These vital cells have been also reported to be infected by the Zika virus (Dhiman et al., 2019). As a result of nerve damage, Schwann cells may trans-differentiate into proliferative cells, which are susceptible to producing inflammatory molecules that aid in myelin removal by macrophages and have the ability to trigger local immunological responses. It has been found that some important inflammatory molecules, such as tumour necrosis factor (TNF)α, interleukin (IL)-1β, IL-6, Leukemia inhibitory factor (LIF), IL-12, and IL-18, are produced by Schwann cells in response to inflammation caused by Zika virus (Oh et al., 2017).

7.3 CONCLUDING REMARKS

Previously, ZIKV was thought to be a comparatively harmless viral infection. Nevertheless, with its increasing prevalence, there is now significant concern, as this infection is coupled with some severe neurological impairments, such as GBS and microcephaly. The human health and financial consequences associated with this outbreak cannot be overestimated. The risk of neuropathies due to ZIKV infection is a significant worry for societies with a higher birth rate, and the physical, financial, and psychiatric difficulties faced by people are aggravated by deteriorating healthcare systems that are unable to effectively cope with existing epidemics. At present, there is no vaccine for ZIKV; thus, developing novel treatment techniques should be one of the top goals at this time. All medications that might be used during pregnancy must be safe. Meanwhile, urgent measures must involve the advancement of better and faster screening methods as well as efficient vector control approaches. There is a requirement to regulate the environmental factors that are responsible for spread of this infection, as it is evident that the increase in human population, rapid urbanisation, industrialisation, and a paucity of efficient prevention strategies are among critical characteristics that have contributed to the establishment of the Zika virus. It is also important to understand and study numerous other aspects of infection that lead to the increased occurrence of impaired neurodevelopment.

CONFLICT OF INTEREST

No conflict of interest

ACKNOWLEDGMENTS

Ishfaq A Ahanger acknowledges the facilities and support at CIRBSc, Jamia Millia Islamia, New Delhi. Shah Ubaid-ullah is thankful to Mr. Sheikh M Saleem, Head Biotechnology, ICSC, Srinagar for his encouragement and extending internet facility for this work.

REFERENCES

Abbink, Peter, Kathryn E Stephenson, and Dan H Barouch. 2018. "Zika virus vaccines." *Nature Reviews in Microbiology* 16(10):594–600.

Agumadu, Vivian C, and Kamleshun Ramphul. 2018. "Zika virus: A review of literature." *Cureus* 10(7). e3025. DOI10.7759/cureus.3025

Ahanger, Ishfaq Ahmad. 2021. "The pathogenesis and complications associated with autism spectrum disorder and Alzheimer's disease: A comparative study." Springer Singapore. https://books.google.co.in/books?id=FI5_zgEACAAJ:325.

Ahanger, Ishfaq Ahmad, Sania Bashir, Zahoor Ahmad Parray, Mohamed F Alajmi, Afzal Hussain, Faizan Ahmad, Md Imtaiyaz Hassan, Asimul Islam, and Anurag Sharma. 2021. "Rationalizing the role of monosodium glutamate in the protein aggregation through biophysical approaches: Potential impact on neurodegeneration." *Frontiers in Neuroscience* 15: 636454. doi: 10.3389/fnins.2021.636454 15.

Ahanger, Ishfaq Ahmad, Zahoor Ahmad Parray, Khalida Nasreen, Faizan Ahmad, Md Imtaiyaz Hassan, Asimul Islam, and Anurag Sharma. 2021. "Heparin accelerates the protein aggregation via the downhill polymerization mechanism: Multi-spectroscopic studies to delineate the implications on proteinopathies." *ACS Omega* 6(3):2328–2339.

Anaya, Juan-Manuel, Carolina Ramirez-Santana, Ignacio Salgado-Castaneda, Christopher Chang, Aftab Ansari, and M Eric Gershwin. 2016. "Zika virus and neurologic autoimmunity: The putative role of gangliosides." *BMC Medicine* 14(1):1–3.

Asad, Hina, and David O Carpenter. 2018. "Effects of climate change on the spread of zika virus: A public health threat." *Reviews on Environmental Health* 33(1):31–42.

Basarab, Marina, Conor Bowman, Emma J Aarons, and Ian Cropley. 2016. "Zika virus." *BMJ: British Medical Journal* 352: i1049. doi:10.1136/bmj.i1049.

Bashir, Sania, Ishfaq Ahmad Ahanger, Anas Shamsi, Mohamed F Alajmi, Afzal Hussain, Hani Choudhry, Faizan Ahmad, Md Hassan, and Asimul Islam. 2021. "Trehalose restrains the fibril load towards α-lactalbumin aggregation and halts fibrillation in a concentration-dependent manner." *Biomolecules* 11(3):414.

Beaver, Jacob T, Nadia Lelutiu, Rumi Habib, and Ioanna Skountzou. 2018. "Evolution of two major Zika virus lineages: Implications for pathology, immune response, and vaccine development." *Frontiers in Immunology* 9:1640.

Ben-Zeev, B, C Hoffman, D Lev, N Watemberg, G Malinger, N Brand, and T Lerman-Sagie. 2003. "Progressive cerebellocerebral atrophy: A new syndrome with microcephaly, mental retardation, and spastic quadriplegia." *Journal of Medical Genetics* 40(8):e96–e96.

Brady, Oliver J, Aaron Osgood-Zimmerman, Nicholas J Kassebaum, Sarah E Ray, Valdelaine EM de Araújo, Aglaêr A da Nóbrega, Livia CV Frutuoso, Roberto CR Lecca, Antony Stevens, and Bruno Zoca de Oliveira. 2019. "The association between Zika virus infection and microcephaly in Brazil 2015–2017: An observational analysis of over 4 million births." *PLOS Medicine* 16(3):e1002755.

Cao-Lormeau, Van-Mai, Alexandre Blake, Sandrine Mons, Stéphane Lastère, Claudine Roche, Jessica Vanhomwegen, Timothée Dub, Laure Baudouin, Anita Teissier, and Philippe Larre. 2016. "Guillain–Barré syndrome outbreak associated with Zika virus infection in French Polynesia: A case-control study." *The Lancet* 387(10027):1531–1539.

Cao-Lormeau, Van-Mai, Claudine Roche, Anita Teissier, Emilie Robin, Anne-Laure Berry, Henri-Pierre Mallet, Amadou Alpha Sall, and Didier Musso. 2014. "Zika virus, French Polynesia, South Pacific, 2013." *Emerging Infectious Diseases* 20(6):1085.

Cardoso, Cristiane W, Igor AD Paploski, Mariana Kikuti, Moreno S Rodrigues, Monaise MO Silva, Gubio S Campos, Silvia I Sardi, Uriel Kitron, Mitermayer G Reis, and Guilherme S Ribeiro. 2015. "Outbreak of exanthematous illness associated with Zika, chikungunya, and dengue viruses, Salvador, Brazil." *Emerging Infectious Diseases* 21(12):2274.

Carlson, Colin J, Eric R Dougherty, and Wayne Getz. 2016. "An ecological assessment of the pandemic threat of Zika virus." *PLOS Neglected Tropical Diseases* 10(8):e0004968.

Carod-Artal, Francisco Javier. 2018. "Neurological complications of Zika virus infection." *Expert Review of Anti-Infective Therapy* 16(5):399–410.

Chala, Bayissa, and Workineh Torben. 2018. "An epidemiological trend of urogenital schistosomiasis in Ethiopia." *Frontiers in Public Health* 6:60.

de Araújo, Thalia Velho Barreto, Ricardo Arraes de Alencar Ximenes, Demócrito de Barros Miranda-Filho, Wayner Vieira Souza, Ulisses Ramos Montarroyos, Ana Paula Lopes de Melo, Sandra Valongueiro, Cynthia Braga, Sinval Pinto Brandão Filho, and Marli Tenório Cordeiro. 2018. "Association between microcephaly, Zika virus infection, and other risk factors in Brazil: final report of a case-control study." *The Lancet Infectious Diseases* 18(3):328–336.

De Koning, TJ. 2006. "Treatment with amino acids in serine deficiency disorders." *Journal of Inherited Metabolic Disease* 29(2–3):347–351.

Dhiman, Gaurav, Rachy Abraham, and Diane E Griffin. 2019. "Human Schwann cells are susceptible to infection with Zika and yellow fever viruses, but not dengue virus." *Scientific Reports* 9(1):1–11.

Egloff, Charles, Christelle Vauloup-Fellous, Olivier Picone, Laurent Mandelbrot, and Pierre Roques. 2020. "Evidence and possible mechanisms of rare maternal-fetal transmission of SARS-CoV-2." *Journal of Clinical Virology* 128:104447.

Faheem, Muhammad, Muhammad Imran Naseer, Mahmood Rasool, Adeel G Chaudhary, Taha A Kumosani, Asad Muhammad Ilyas, Peter Natesan Pushparaj, Farid Ahmed, Hussain A Algahtani, and Mohammad H Al-Qahtani. 2015. "Molecular genetics of human primary microcephaly: An overview." *BMC Medical Genomics* 8(1):1–11.

Faye, Oumar, Ousmane Faye, Anne Dupressoir, Manfred Weidmann, Mady Ndiaye, and Amadou Alpha Sall. 2008. "One-step RT-PCR for detection of Zika virus." *Journal of Clinical Virology* 43(1):96–101.

Faye, Oumar, Caio CM Freire, Atila Iamarino, Ousmane Faye, Juliana Velasco C de Oliveira, Mawlouth Diallo, Paolo M A Zanotto, Amadou Alpha Sall. 2014. "Molecular evolution of Zika virus during its emergence in the 20th century." *PLOS Neglected Tropical Diseases* 8(1):e2636.

Ferreira, Priscila Gonçalves, Blanka Tesla, Elvira Cynthia Alves Horácio, Laila Alves Nahum, Melinda Ann Brindley, Tiago Antônio de Oliveira Mendes, and Courtney Cuinn Murdock. 2020. "Temperature dramatically shapes mosquito gene expression with consequences for mosquito–Zika virus interactions." *Frontiers in Microbiology* 11:901.

Gobillot, Theodore A, Daryl Humes, Amit Sharma, Caroline Kikawa, and Julie Overbaugh. 2020. "The robust restriction of zika virus by type-I interferon in A549 cells varies by viral lineage and is not determined by IFITM3." *Viruses* 12(5):503.

Kostyuchenko, Victor A, Elisa XY Lim, Shuijun Zhang, Guntur Fibriansah, Thiam-Seng Ng, Justin SG Ooi, Jian Shi, and Shee-Mei Lok. 2016. "Structure of the thermally stable Zika virus." *Nature* 533(7603):425–428.

Kraemer, Moritz UG, Marianne E Sinka, Kirsten A Duda, Adrian QN Mylne, Freya M Shearer, Christopher M Barker, Chester G Moore, Roberta G Carvalho, Giovanini E Coelho, and Wim Van Bortel. 2015. "The global distribution of the arbovirus vectors Aedes aegypti and Ae. albopictus." *eLife* 4:e08347.

Krauer, Fabienne, Maurane Riesen, Ludovic Reveiz, Olufemi T Oladapo, Ruth Martínez-Vega, Teegwende V Porgo, Anina Haefliger, Nathalie J Broutet, Nicola Low, and WHO Zika Causality Working Group. 2017. "Zika virus infection as a cause of congenital brain abnormalities and Guillain–Barré syndrome: Systematic review." *PLOS Medicine* 14(1):e1002203.

Meaney-Delman, Dana, Titilope Oduyebo, Kara ND Polen, Jennifer L White, Andrea M Bingham, Sally A Slavinski, Lea Heberlein-Larson, Kirsten St George, Jennifer L Rakeman, and Susan Hills. 2016. "Prolonged detection of Zika virus RNA in pregnant women." *Obstetrics & Gynecology* 128(4):724–730.

Messina, Jane P, Moritz UG Kraemer, Oliver J Brady, David M Pigott, Freya M Shearer, Daniel J Weiss, Nick Golding, Corrine W Ruktanonchai, Peter W Gething, and Emily Cohn. 2016. "Mapping global environmental suitability for Zika virus." *eLife* 5:e15272.

Monaghan, Andrew J, Cory W Morin, Daniel F Steinhoff, Olga Wilhelmi, Mary Hayden, Dale A Quattrochi, Michael Reiskind, Alun L Lloyd, Kirk Smith, and Chris A Schmidt. 2016. "On the seasonal occurrence and abundance of the Zika virus vector mosquito Aedes aegypti in the contiguous United States." *PLOS Currents* 8. doi: 10.1371/currents.outbreaks.50dfc7f46798675fc63e7d7da563da76

Monel, Blandine, Alex A Compton, Timothée Bruel, Sonia Amraoui, Julien Burlaud-Gaillard, Nicolas Roy, Florence Guivel-Benhassine, Françoise Porrot, Pierre Génin, and Laurent Meertens. 2017. "Zika virus induces massive cytoplasmic vacuolization and paraptosis-like death in infected cells." *The EMBO Journal* 36(12):1653–1668.

Mooney, Chris. 2016. "The hidden environmental factors behind the spread of Zika and other devastating diseases." *The Washington Post* 3. https://www.washingtonpost.com/news/energy-environment/wp/2016/02/03/the-hidden-environmental-factors-behind-the-spread-of-zika-and-other-deadly-diseases/

Mumtaz, Noreen, Jeroen JA van Kampen, Chantal BEM Reusken, Charles AB Boucher, and Marion PG Koopmans. 2016. "Zika virus: Where is the treatment?" *Current Treatment Options in Infectious Diseases* 8(3):208–211.

Nobuhiro, Yuki, and HP Hartung. 2012. "Guillain–Barré syndrome." *New England Journal of Medicine* 366(24):2294–2304.

Oehler, Erwan, L Watrin, P Larre, I Leparc-Goffart, S Lastere, F Valour, L Baudouin, HP Mallet, D Musso, and F Ghawche. 2014. "Zika virus infection complicated by Guillain-Barre syndrome–case report, French Polynesia, December 2013." *Eurosurveillance* 19(9):20720.

Oh, Yohan, Feiran Zhang, Yaqing Wang, Emily M Lee, Young Choi, Hotae Lim, Fahimeh Mirakhori, Ronghua Li, Luoxiu Huang, and Tianlei Xu. 2017. "Zika virus directly infects peripheral neurons and induces cell death." *Nature Neuroscience* 20(9):1209–1212.

Ornelas, Alice MM, Paula Pezzuto, Paola P Silveira, Fabiana O Melo, Thales A Ferreira, Patricia S Oliveira-Szejnfeld, Jeime I Leal, Melania MR Amorim, Stuart Hamilton, and William D Rawlinson. 2017. "Immune activation in amniotic fluid from Zika virus–associated microcephaly." *Annals of Neurology* 81(1):152–156.

Parra, Beatriz, Jairo Lizarazo, Jorge A Jiménez-Arango, Andrés F Zea-Vera, Guillermo González-Manrique, José Vargas, Jorge A Angarita, Gonzalo Zuñiga, Reydmar Lopez-Gonzalez, and Cindy L Beltran. 2016. "Guillain–Barré syndrome associated with Zika virus infection in Colombia." *New England Journal of Medicine* 375(16):1513–1523.

Rather, Irfan A, Jameel B Lone, Vivek K Bajpai, and Yong-Ha Park. 2017. "Zika virus infection during pregnancy and congenital abnormalities." *Frontiers in Microbiology* 8:581.

Reyna-Villasmil, Eduardo, Geraldine López-Sánchez, and Joel Santos-Bolívar. 2016. "Guillain-Barre syndrome due to Zika virus during pregnancy." *Medicina Clinica* 146(7):331–332.

Rodríguez-Barraquer, Isabel, Henrik Salje, Justin Lessler, and Derek AT Cummings. 2016. "Predicting intensities of Zika infection and microcephaly using transmission intensities of other arboviruses." *bioRxiv* 041095; doi: https://doi.org/10.1101/041095.

Ropper, Allan H. 1992. "The Guillain–Barré syndrome." *New England Journal of Medicine* 326(17):1130–1136.

Saumya, Kumar Udit, Kundlik Gadhave, Amit Kumar, and Rajanish Giri. 2020. "Zika virus capsid anchor forms cytotoxic amyloid-like fibrils." *bioRxiv* 041095; doi: https://doi.org/10.1101/041095.

Schwartz, David A. 2017. "The origins and emergence of Zika virus, the newest torch infection: What's old is new again." *Archives of Pathology & Laboratory Medicine* 141(1):18–25.

Shi, Yi, and George F Gao. 2017. "Structural biology of the Zika virus." *Trends in Biochemical Sciences* 42(6):443–456.

Taybeh, Noura. 2020. "Examining zika virus: Transmission, diagnosis, treatment, and prevention." *BU Well* 5(1):14.

Tunali, Merve, Alexandro André Radin, Selma Başıbüyük, Anwar Musah, Iuri Valerio Graciano Borges, Orhan Yenigun, Aisha Aldosery, Patty Kostkova, Wellington P Dos Santos, and Tiago Massoni. 2021. "A review exploring the overarching burden of Zika virus with emphasis on epidemiological case studies from Brazil." *Environmental Science & Pollution Research International* 28(40):55952–55966.

Valente, Ana Paula, and Adolfo Henrique Moraes. 2019. "Zika virus proteins at an atomic scale: How does structural biology help us to understand and develop vaccines and drugs against Zika virus infection?" *Journal of Venomous Animals & Toxins Including Tropical Diseases* 25: e20190013. doi: 10.1590/1678-9199-JVAT ITD-2019-0013.

Valentine, Gregory, Lucila Marquez, and Mohan Pammi. 2016. "Zika virus-associated microcephaly and eye lesions in the newborn." *Journal of the Pediatric Infectious Diseases Society* 5(3):323–328.

Van den Berg, B, C Walgaard, J Drenthen, C Fokke, BC Jacobs, and PA van Doorn. 2014. "Guillain–Barré syndrome: Pathogenesis, diagnosis, treatment and prognosis." *Nature Reviews Neurology* 10(8):469–482.

Viennet, Elvina, Francesca D Frentiu, Craig R Williams, Gina Mincham, Cassie C Jansen, Brian L Montgomery, Robert LP Flower, and Helen M Faddy. 2020. "Estimation of mosquito-borne and sexual transmission of Zika virus in Australia: Risks to blood transfusion safety." *PLOS Neglected Tropical Diseases* 14(7):e0008438.

Wang, Zhaoyang, Peigang Wang, and Jing An. 2016. "Zika virus and Zika fever." *Virologica Sinica* 31(2):103–109.

Wen, Zhexing, Hongjun Song, and Guo-li Ming. 2017. "How does Zika virus cause microcephaly?" *Genes & Development* 31(9):849–861.

Wilke, André BB, John C Beier, and Giovanni Benelli. 2019. "Complexity of the relationship between global warming and urbanization–an obscure future for predicting increases in vector-borne infectious diseases." *Current Opinion in Insect Science* 35:1–9.

Županc, Tatjana Avšic, and Miroslav Petrovec. 2016. "Zika: An old virus with a new face." *Slovenian Journal of Public Health* 55(4):228.

8 Emerging Contaminants in the Environment and Their Linkage with COVID-19

Majid Peyravi and Marjan Sadat Mirmasoomi

CONTENTS

8.1 Introduction 117
8.2 Emerging Contaminants 118
8.2.1 Pharmaceutical Industries 119
8.2.2 Personal Care Products 120
8.2.3 Pesticides 120
8.3 Treatment Methods for Emerging Contaminants 121
8.3.1 Adsorptive Membranes 121
8.3.1.1 Homogeneous Membranes 122
8.3.1.2 Mixed Matrix Membranes 122
8.3.1.3 Composite Membranes 123
8.3.2 Photocatalytic Membranes 123
8.3.3 Membrane Bioreactors 124
8.3.4 Molecularly Imprinted Membranes 125
8.3.5 Affinity Membranes 125
8.4 Conclusion 126
References 126

8.1 INTRODUCTION

Water is an essential natural resource for humans and many production industries (Rathi et al., 2021). In recent years, the development of various industries and technologies and the increase in population growth have led to the production of complex chemicals and toxic compounds that have caused severe pollution and the lack of healthy water (Mansoori et al., 2020). Pollution of water resources is a worldwide problem that threatens the ecosystem and health of humans and other organisms (Litchfield et al., 2020).

Water demand is increasing due to climate change, population growth, economic development, and environmental degradation (Rathi et al., 2021). Also,

DOI: 10.1201/9781003288732-8

the introduction of contaminated water into the body of humans and other living organisms causes severe damage to them and various diseases. For instance, heavy metals are one of the emerging toxic pollutants whose continuous consumption by humans causes multiple conditions such as renal damage, hypertension, emphysema, and skeletal malformation in fetuses (Chong et al., 2019).

Emerging contaminants consist of personal care products, human and veterinary pharmaceuticals, pesticides, plasticisers, and different industrial additives that have become a severe environmental and societal concern given their toxicity (Rathi et al., 2021; Liu et al., 2021). Hence, emerging or newly identified contaminants in water resources and the environment can threaten wastewater and water quality and cause the emergence and proliferation of diseases affecting humans and all living organisms (Rathi et al., 2021; Patz et al., 2000). Therefore, researchers have been raising awareness of new contaminants that require treatment and removal, especially because of the coronavirus (COVID 19) pandemic, which caused the increased production and consumption of emerging pollutants of unknown and complex nature.

To address these problems, the treatment methods for water resources and their reuse have attracted considerable attention. Conventional contaminant removal techniques include filtration, adsorption, ion exchange, electrochemical treatment, advanced oxidation processes, and multistep coagulation and flocculation (Vo et al., 2020). However, these methods have disadvantages, such as high energy consumption, operational problems, and low economic benefits (Mansoori et al., 2020). In addition, another problem with some of these methods is the risk of secondary contaminants (Wen et al., 2013). Among these methods, the membrane process is recognised as an effective method for eliminating contaminants from water sources. This technique's advantages include low energy consumption, uncomplicated process, relatively good economic efficiency, and zero sludge production.

Emerging pollutants are consumed in large quantities daily and discharged into rivers and wastewater in concentrations ranging from nanograms to micrograms per litre (Tran et al., 2018). Considering the low concentration range of pollutants, using new processes and integrating two or more wastewater treatment processes can be a good candidate for effectively and efficiently removing emerging pollutants. Thus, this chapter is oriented to emerging contaminants and their removal methods using different effective membrane processes and combining water and wastewater treatment processes with membrane filtration using adsorptive membranes, photocatalytic membranes, membrane bioreactors, molecularly imprinted membranes, and affinity membranes.

8.2 EMERGING CONTAMINANTS

Detecting so-called emerging or newly identified contaminants has attracted worldwide attention due to their toxic and carcinogenic effects on living bodies. Yet, it is challenging to remove emerging pollutants from water, sewage, and the environment due to their continuous emission and very low concentration (in the microgram or nanogram per litre range) (Taheran et al., 2018). Furthermore, these pollutants may have adverse effects on human and marine organisms in low concentrations (Rathi et al., 2021). In addition, the chemical properties of these contaminants, such as solubility, molecular weight, polarity, and electric charge, are different, making them difficult to remove using conventional treatment systems (Verlichhi et al., 2012). Research has shown that emerging pollutants are produced in pharmaceuticals, personal care products, pesticides, plasticisers, surfactants, food additives, wood preservatives, laundry detergents, disinfectants, flame retardants, and other industrial additives, but the amount of pollutants produced by the pharmaceutical industry, personal care products, and pesticides is greater.

8.2.1 Pharmaceutical Industries

In recent years, the use of pharmaceutical compounds and vaccines (especially due to the coronavirus pandemic) has increased due to antimicrobial resistance (AMR) (Mandal et al., 2019). Although pharmaceutical compounds are present only in small amounts in water and wastewater sources, they are dangerous and disturbing (Rathi et al., 2021). Research by Cetecioglu et al. shows that pharmaceutical wastewater, entering water mainly from various sources such as hospitals, veterinary clinics, households, and drug production facilities, has high chemical oxygen demand (COD) (4,410–40,000 mg/L) with high concentrations of nitrogen compounds (Mandal et al., 2019; Behera et al., 2011; Cetecioglu et al., 2015). These pharmaceuticals include antibiotics, hormonal drugs, vaccines, antacids, clofibric acid, steroids, antidepressants, analgesics, salicylic acid, anti-inflammatory drugs, propranolol, antipyretics, beta-blockers, fluoxetine, nitroglycerin, and lipid-lowering drugs (Rathi et al., 2021). Furthermore, the persistence of pharmaceutical products in water and wastewater sources is accompanied by hormonal imbalances that cause various diseases such as decreased fertility, reproductive impairments, and breast and testosterone-related cancers (Dhanger et al., 2020; Ahmed et al., 2015).

Antibiotics are chemical drugs used to stop the growth of bacteria or kill them. Antibiotics are widely used to prevent and treat human and animal diseases. Commonly used antibiotics in human practice are fluoroquinolones, macrolides, and aminoglycosides (Milic et al., 2013). The most common antibiotics used in veterinary medicine to treat and control infectious diseases such as mastitis, enteritis, peritonitis, and pneumonia are penicillins, tetracyclines, and macrolides (Milic et al., 2013). Among all emerging contaminants, one of the major concerns is the presence of antibiotics in water sources, which can lead to the spreading of antibiotic resistance genes in bacteria (Dhanger et al., 2020; Ahmed et al., 2015).

Another concern is the increasing use of drugs and vaccines against the new virus. On 13 March 2020, the coronavirus (COVID-19) was declared a pandemic by the World Health Organization (WHO) and is still considered a global crisis. Due to this pandemic, emerging pathogens can be transmitted through human waste, agriculture, animals, hospital effluents, or surface water, which can negatively impact humans and the environment (Cheval et al., 2020).

8.2.2 Personal Care Products

Personal care products are a variety of chemicals used to improve, maintain, and promote health, beauty, and personal hygiene. Unfortunately, increasing the daily consumption of skin care products causes a large volume of them to be released into the air (Rathi et al., 2020). Personal care products cover tranquillisers, stimulants, fragrances, sunscreen agents, cosmetics, skin products, hair care products, cleaning products, and shampoos that contain toxic and complex compounds (polydimethylsiloxane, nano titanium dioxide, butylated hydroxylanisole), insect repellents, microplastics, butylated hydroxytoluene, disinfectants (triclosan and triclocarban), fragrances (galaxolide, tonalite, celestolide, and phantolide), and preservatives (diethyl phthalate, nano zinc oxide, benzophenone, parabens, octinoxate methoxycinnamate, and butylparaben) (Dhanirama et al., 2012; Montes-Grajales, 2017; Miege et al., 2009). These pollutants reach the aquatic environment through sewage by directly discharging raw or treated water (Ricky and Shanthakumar, 2022). Furthermore, the presence of these compounds in water sources causes diseases such as obesity, diabetes, hypertension, subfertility, and endometriosis (Ferguson et al., 2017).

8.2.3 Pesticides

Toxic chemicals used in agricultural and non-agricultural areas to reduce or prevent damage from insects, weeds, fungi, and other dangerous pests are called pesticides. Traditional and environmentally friendly pesticides are considered for plant growth and increasing crop productivity (Liang et al., 2022). However, most pesticides are stable in soil, atmosphere, and water, remain intact for a long time, and enter the human body and other living organisms, endangering the ecosystem and disturbing the ecological balance (Gilden et al., 2010).

Human exposure to pesticides can occur through direct means like contact or ingestion of food and inhalation. However, once in the body, these pollutants can cause various diseases such as asthma and chronic obstructive pulmonary disease (COPD), cardiovascular diseases such as atherosclerosis and coronary artery disease, chronic nephropathies, autoimmune diseases like systemic lupus erythematosus and rheumatoid arthritis, and chronic fatigue syndrome (Lorthuraj et al., 2022).

With improper use of different pesticides and increasing consumption of healthier food products, detecting pesticide residues in aquatic and wastewater environments is controversial. So far, most diagnostic methods have included chromatography, spectrophotometry, and rapid detection methodology (Liang et al., 2022).

Based on targeted organisms, pesticides are classified into herbicides, fungicides, insecticides, nematicides, and avicides. In addition, pesticides can be divided into two categories: traditional and environmentally friendly (Lian et al., 2022).

Traditional pesticides based on chemical structure include groups of organochlorine pesticides (OCPs), organophosphate pesticides (OPPs), pyrethroid pesticides, and carbamate. About 45% of the pesticides used worldwide are organophosphates. The use of 140 types of organophosphates has been reported worldwide, causing severe damage to soil and water and resulting in more than 200,000 deaths per year. Organophosphates may be in the form of a pale yellow, pale brown oily liquid or white crystals. Most of them are insecticides, and a few of them are fungicides and herbicides (Liang et al., 2022; Ojha et al., 2013).

Environmentally friendly pesticides contain biologically active substances or substances such as *Bacillus thuringiensis*, plant-based matrine, and toosendanin. Therefore, the demand for their use is increasing day by day. These pesticides are quickly degraded in agricultural products and soil and do not harm the environment. One of the most widely used pesticides is *Bacillus thuringiensis*, which protects agricultural products against pests such as *Lepidoptera*, *Coleoptera*, and *Diptera*. Compared with traditional pesticides, these pesticides are environmentally friendly and less toxic to humans (Liang et al., 2022; Ramli et al., 2018).

8.3 TREATMENT METHODS FOR EMERGING CONTAMINANTS

Traditional wastewater treatment methods cannot remove emerging contaminants, and additional treatment is required to remove them. Therefore, methods such as adsorption, advanced oxidation, and membrane processes are used as additional treatment processes. In addition, a combination of these processes is used to remove emerging contaminants, including adsorptive membrane, photocatalytic membrane, and molecularly imprinted membrane, as explained in the following subsections.

8.3.1 Adsorptive Membranes

The adsorptive membrane was discovered in the 1980s (Heitner-Wirguin, 1996). Recently, adsorptive membranes have attracted much attention for removing emerging contaminants from aqueous solutions due to two simultaneous advantages: the adsorption process and membrane separation.

Compared with standard adsorption and membrane filtration methods, adsorptive membranes have some advantages, such as low internal diffusion resistance, fast kinetics, adsorption/desorption rates, low operating pressure, high permeability flux, and increased removal rates (Huang et al., 2020; Hao et al., 2021; Adam et al., 2019). However, large-scale industrial adsorption membranes may have high process costs, low adsorption capacity, and limited reusability. Moreover, one of the most important points about adsorption membranes is their ability to regenerate and reuse adsorbents. Therefore, the adsorbents used in adsorptive membranes should be chemically stable and reusable so that these types of membranes become more economical and eco-friendly (Vo et al., 2020).

In the adsorption process, the contaminants adhere to the adsorbent by physical or chemical interactions. The physical adsorption process is performed by van der Waals force, and in the chemical adsorption, a chemical reaction is performed between the adsorbent molecules and the contaminants (Autumn et al., 2000). In an adsorptive membrane, when contaminants come in contact with adsorbents, functional groups on the surface and pore walls of the membrane selectively adsorb the pollutants. In general, in physical adsorption, less contact time is required between the adsorbent and the pollutant, and in chemical adsorption, due to the strong chemical bonding of the adsorbent with contaminants, more contact time is needed to reach equilibrium (Vo et al., 2020).

Adsorptive membranes are classified based on structure as follows: homogeneous membranes (inorganic or organic), mixed matrix membranes, and composite membranes (surface composite or sandwich composite) (Hao et al., 2021).

8.3.1.1 Homogeneous Membranes

Homogeneous adsorptive membranes are divided into two categories, organic and inorganic membranes, both of which are single-phase (Hao et al., 2021).

8.3.1.1.1 Organic Adsorptive Membranes

This type of membrane uses natural, renewable, and biodegradable materials resulting from the presence of nitrogen and oxygen in their chemical structure (Qalyoubi et al., 2021). Using organic materials in adsorptive membranes can remove a wide range of contaminants; for instance, chitosan, which has large numbers of amine functional groups, is suitable for removing various pollutants (Adam et al., 2019; Qalyoubi et al., 2021). It is a highly capable substance whose removal function depends on the potential of amine functional groups (Hao et al., 2021).

8.3.1.1.2 Inorganic Adsorptive Membranes

Inorganic adsorptive membranes use synthetic materials that are easier to regenerate than organic materials due to their stability (Bhave et al., 2012; Verweij, 2012). Common materials used in inorganic adsorption membranes consist of oxides or metals such as Al_2O_3, TiO_2, SiO_2, MgO, RuO_2, and Si_3N_4 (Hao et al., 2021).

8.3.1.2 Mixed Matrix Membranes

The specific adsorbents are dispersed at the nanometre level in the polymeric matrix; hence the name mixed matrix membranes (Vinh-Thang and Serge Kaliaguine, 2013). Mixed matrix membranes have been widely studied to eliminate emerging contaminants from water and wastewater. These membranes are easy to prepare, but disadvantages include lower adsorption capacity and longer adsorption equilibrium time (Qalyoubi, 2021).

Adsorbents used in mixed matrix membranes can be organic, inorganic, inorganic-organic, and biological, depending on the contaminant type and its application (Hao et al., 2021). For instance, Mukherjee et al. made a mixed matrix membrane using polysulfone and graphene oxide and removed the heavy metals Pb^{2+}, Cu^{2+}, Cd^{2+}, and Cr^{6+} with adsorption capacity of 79, 75, 68 and 154 mg/g, respectively (Mukherjee et al., 2016).

8.3.1.3 Composite Membranes

Composite membranes consist of two layers made of different materials, divided into two categories of surface and sandwich composite membranes based on the location of the absorbent layer.

8.3.1.3.1 Surface Composite Membranes

In this type of membrane, due to the surface membrane adsorbent, the adsorption rate is better because the membrane is in direct contact with the solution and contaminants (Mansoori et al., 2020).

8.3.1.3.2 Sandwich Composite Membranes

In sandwich membranes, the adsorbent layer is located between the support and surface layers. The advantages of this type of membrane are high strength and stability due to the penetration of the surface layer solution into the substrate's pores and reduction of fouling due to the asymmetric structure of the surface layer (Mansoori et al., 2020).

8.3.2 Photocatalytic Membranes

Photocatalysis, an environmentally friendly advanced oxidation process, has become an emerging technology that can degrade many organic and toxic pollutants in water and wastewater sources. By activating a photon, a photocatalyst is activated. The photocatalytic process consists of four stages: absorption of light with desirable energy (suitable with catalyst), separation of electron–hole pair, reactant adsorption onto active sites, main reaction, and desorption of ultimate products (Darbandi et al., 2019; Kıranşan et al., 2015; Khataee et al., 2019; Nasrollahi et al., 2021). For example, photocatalysts are activated by absorbing radiation on the surface of metal oxides and transferring electrons from the valence band to the conduction band. As a result, electron–hole pairs formed with oxygen and hydroxyl groups in water react to constitute various reactive oxygen species (ROSs) such as •OH, $O2^{-}$•, and H_2O_2 (Shi et al., 2019; Zheng et al., 2017).

Semiconductors such as TiO_2, ZnO, CuO, Fe_2O_3, CNTs/g-C_3N_4, and rGo/g-C_3N_4 are used in the photocatalytic process (Shi et al., 2019). Titanium dioxide (TiO_2) has received more attention from researchers due to its multi-faceted functional properties such as good chemical and thermal stability, high structural stability, excellent catalytic properties, and low price compared with other semiconductors (Tong et al., 2012; Ganiyu et al., 2015).

Photocatalysis has advantages, such as converting toxic pollutants into harmless substances like water and carbon dioxide, simple working conditions, high process efficiency, and low cost (Shrama et al., 2008; Lhomme et al., 2008; Lee et al., 2013; Oancea et al., 2008; Koe, 2020). However, research has demonstrated that the reasons for the non-industrialisation of the photocatalysis process are low use of visible light, the low migration ability of the photo-generated electrons and holes, and fast charge recombination (Judd, 2010). In addition, it is difficult to separate and recycle catalysts from purified water, and photocatalytic membranes can be used to solve this problem (Argurio et al., 2018).

Photocatalytic membranes combine both processes of photocatalyst and membrane filtration. Photocatalytic membranes have demonstrated high effectiveness in emerging pollutant removal from wastewater sources. Photocatalytic membranes perform better than the photocatalyst process because they can separate the photocatalyst from the treated effluent. They also have more advantages than the membrane process because they can destroy contaminants by producing oxygen-reactive radicals under light irradiation and prevent membrane fouling (Molinari et al., 2002).

The most famous and widely used photocatalytic membranes are photocatalytic membrane reactors (PMRs). Photocatalytic reactors are multifunctional membrane reactors created by combining a catalytic (photocatalytic) reaction with a membrane process. PMRs have become an attractive option over conventional photo reactors due to several advantages, including placing the photocatalyst in the reaction environment using the membrane, separating products and catalysts simultaneously from the reaction environment, and inhibiting the retention time of molecules in the reactor (Zhang et al., 2016). This reduces energy consumption and operating costs and increases catalyst reusability and process stability (Zheng et al., 2017).

Photocatalytic reactors are divided into two categories based on the location of the photocatalysts relative to the membranes: (i) slurry PMRs (PMRs with solubilised or suspended photocatalyst in the reaction mixture); and (ii) immobilised PMRs (PMRs with photocatalyst fixed in/on a membrane) (Mozia, 2010).

In PMRs with suspended photocatalysts, the active surface available for the solution is much higher than when the photocatalyst is fixed on the membrane because by placing the photocatalyst on the membrane, a large amount of active surface is reduced, which causes active light loss (Li et al., 2015).

8.3.3 Membrane Bioreactors

Membrane bioreactors result from a combination of biological treatment processes, such as activated sludge, with a direct solid–liquid separation by a membrane filtration unit, with many commercial and industrial applications. In membrane bioreactors, microorganisms such as bacteria, algae, and fungi are located in the feed solution and contribute to water purification by physical retention and microbial degradation of contaminants (Li et al., 2015). Furthermore, microfiltration and ultrafiltration membranes are primarily applied in various modules and configurations, the most useful of which are flat-sheet and hollow fibre membrane modules (Li et al., 2011; Nunes et al., 2001). Membrane bioreactors have advantages over conventional treatment methods, such as the small footprint size of the treatment plant, excellent effluent quality, optimal disinfection capacity, lower sludge production, and higher volume loading (Ahmed et al., 2017; Jud and Simon, 2010). However, through time, the performance of membrane bioreactors decreases due to membrane fouling (Le-Clech et al., 2006).

MBRs are structurally divided into two categories (Li et al., 2011):

1. Submerged or immersed unit (sMBR)
2. (Side-stream, cross flow) external unit (cfMBR)

The energy requirement in sMBR is less than in cfMBR, but both are effective on an industrial scale in removing contaminants from water and wastewater (Li et al., 2011).

8.3.4 Molecularly Imprinted Membranes

Molecularly imprinted polymers (MIPs) are synthetic polymers that take a model of a specific target molecule until they separate the target molecule with high selectivity (Yoshikawa et al., 2016). In other words, MIPs are artificial receptors to adsorb a particular target molecule (Mukherjee et al., 2016). The advantages of a molecularly imprinted polymer are its cheapness, high temperature and pressure resistance, high stability, physical robustness, and chemical inertness compared with other biological systems (Xu et al., 2004; Huang et al., 2015).

Molecular imprinting is an advanced technology that operates based on a key–lock mechanism; the molecular imprinting technique gives molecular recognition properties to a matrix polymer through polymerisation until it removes specific template molecules (Yoshikawa et al., 2016; Del Blanco et al., 2012; Sobiech et al., 2018).

These techniques have progressed in various fields, including membrane filtration, chromatography, separation and purification of drugs and biological derivatives, chemical sensors, and catalysis (Mukherjee et al., 2016; Del Blanco et al., 2012).

The usage of molecular imprinting for membrane filtration has been investigated since 1962 (Yoshikawa et al., 2016). The imprinting technique, coupled with membrane technology, has exhibited great potential for usage in water purification and wastewater treatment (Mukherjee et al., 2016; Del Blanco et al., 2012). The various configurations of MIMs comprise flat sheets and hollow fibre composites, of which flat-sheet MIMs are the more widely used (Algieri et al., 2014). Flat-sheet MIMs are used to identify several target molecules, such as vitamins (Donato et al., 2010), flavonoids (Trotta et al., 2002), pesticides (Donato et al., 2011), and biomolecules like enzymes and uric acid (Silvestri et al., 2006). Composite MIMs consist of two layers: the support layer is composed of a polymer membrane, and the thin imprinted polymeric layer has molecular recognition properties (Del Blanco et al., 2012).

8.3.5 Affinity Membranes

In this kind of membrane, one specific molecule is placed in an inert matrix for selective removal, and the particular molecule determines its desired molecule from the feed and separates it. These membranes work based on molecular recognition. This operation could solve membrane fouling, a problem of the chromatographic separation method. Among the affinity separation methods, affinity chromatography is employed most frequently. The advantages of this method are high flow rate, low pressure drop, and productivity (Zhou et al., 2001).

8.4 CONCLUSION

Due to the increase of various viruses and microbes, especially coronavirus, toxic pollutants, and complex compounds are being dumped into water and wastewater sources. Emerging pollutants, even in small quantities, have been widely studied due to their severe and toxic environmental effects. These contaminants include different types of pollutants from various industries. Most pollutants come from the pharmaceutical industry, personal care products, and pesticides. These contaminants are challenging to remove with the help of traditional treatment methods. For this reason, the integration of membrane filtration and other purification processes, including adsorptive membranes, photocatalytic membranes, membrane bioreactors, molecularly imprinted membranes, and affinity membranes, is used for the effective removal of emerging pollutants. It should be noted that researchers are still exploring innovations and the use of new technologies in industrial-scale water and wastewater treatment to eliminate these toxic pollutants effectively.

REFERENCES

Adam, Mohd Ridhwan, Siti Khadijah Hubadillah, Mohamad Izrin Mohamad Esham, Mohd. Hafiz Dzarfan Othman, Mukhlis A. Rahman, Ahmad Fauzi Ismail, and Juhana Jaafar. "Adsorptive membranes for heavy metals removal from water." In: *Membrane Separation Principles and Applications*, pp. 361–400. Elsevier, 2019.

Ahmed, Mohammad Boshir, John L. Zhou, Huu Hao Ngo, and Wenshan Guo. "Adsorptive removal of antibiotics from water and wastewater: Progress and challenges." *Science of the Total Environment* 532 (2015): 112–126.

Ahmed, Mohammad Boshir, John L. Zhou, Huu Hao Ngo, Wenshan Guo, Nikolaos S. Thomaidis, and Jiang Xu. "Progress in the biological and chemical treatment technologies for emerging contaminant removal from wastewater: A critical review." *Journal of Hazardous Materials* 323, no. A (2017): 274–298.

Algieri, Catia, Enrico Drioli, Laura Guzzo, and Laura Donato. "Bio-mimetic sensors based on molecularly imprinted membranes." *Sensors* 14, no. 8 (2014): 13863–13912.

Argurio, Pietro, Enrica Fontananova, Raffaele Molinari, and Enrico Drioli. "Photocatalytic membranes in photocatalytic membrane reactors." *Processes* 6, no. 9 (2018): 162.

Autumn, Kellar, Yiching A. Liang, S. Tonia Hsieh, Wolfgang Zesch, Wai Pang Chan, Thomas W. Kenny, Ronald Fearing, and Robert J. Full. "Adhesive force of a single gecko foot-hair." *Nature* 405, no. 6787 (2000): 681–685.

Behera, Shishir Kumar, Hyeong Woo Kim, Jeong-Eun Oh, and Hung-Suck Park. "Occurrence and removal of antibiotics, hormones and several other pharmaceuticals in wastewater treatment plants of the largest industrial city of Korea." *Science of the Total Environment* 409, no. 20 (2011): 4351–4360.

Bhave, Ramesh. *Inorganic Membranes Synthesis, Characteristics and Applications: Synthesis, Characteristics, and Applications*. Springer Science & Business Media, 2012.

Cetecioglu, Zeynep, Bahar Ince, Meritxell Gros, Sara Rodriguez-Mozaz, Damia Barceló, Orhan Ince, and Derin Orhon. "Biodegradation and reversible inhibitory impact of sulfamethoxazole on the utilization of volatile fatty acids during anaerobic treatment of pharmaceutical industry wastewater." *Science of the Total Environment* 536 (2015): 667–674.

Cheval, Sorin, Cristian Mihai Adamescu, Teodoro Georgiadis, Mathew Herrnegger, Adrian Piticar, and David R. Legates. "Observed and potential impacts of the COVID-19 pandemic on the environment." *International Journal of Environmental Research and Public Health* 17, no. 11 (2020): 4140.

Chong, Woon Chan, Yung Lim Choo, Chai Hoon Koo, Yean Ling Pang, and Soon Onn Lai. "Adsorptive membranes for heavy metal removal–A mini review." *AIP Conference Proceedings* 2157, no. 1 (2019): 020005.

Darbandi, Masih, Behrouz Shaabani, Jenny Schneider, Detlef Bahnemann, Peyman Gholami, Alireza Khataee, Pariya Yardani, and Mir Ghasem Hosseini. "TiO_2 nanoparticles with superior hydrogen evolution and pollutant degradation performance." *International Journal of Hydrogen Energy* 44, no. 44 (2019): 24162–24173.

Del Blanco, Samuel García, Laura Donato, and Enrico Drioli. "Development of molecularly imprinted membranes for selective recognition of primary amines in organic medium." *Separation and Purification Technology* 87 (2012): 40–46.

Dhangar, Kiran, and Manish Kumar. "Tricks and tracks in removal of emerging contaminants from the wastewater through hybrid treatment systems: A review." *Science of the Total Environment* 738 (2020): 140320.

Dhanirama, Danelle, Jan Gronow, and Nikolaos Voulvoulis. "Cosmetics as a potential source of environmental contamination in the UK." *Environmental Technology* 33, no. 14 (2012): 1597–1608.

Donato, L., F. Tasselli, and E. Drioli. "Molecularly imprinted membranes with affinity properties for folic acid." *Separation Science and Technology* 45, no. 16 (2010): 2273–2279.

Donato, Laura, Maria Cristina Greco, and Enrico Drioli. "Preparation of molecularly imprinted membranes and evaluation of their performance in the selective recognition of dimethoate." *Desalination and Water Treatment* 30, no. 1–3 (2011): 171–177.

Ferguson, Kelly K., Justin A. Colacino, Ryan C. Lewis, and John D. Meeker. "Personal care product use among adults in NHANES: Associations between urinary phthalate metabolites and phenols and use of mouthwash and sunscreen." *Journal of Exposure Science and Environmental Epidemiology* 27, no. 3 (2017): 326–332.

Ganiyu, Soliu O., Eric D. Van Hullebusch, Marc Cretin, Giovanni Esposito, and Mehmet A. Oturan. "Coupling of membrane filtration and advanced oxidation processes for removal of pharmaceutical residues: A critical review." *Separation and Purification Technology* 156 (2015): 891–914.

Gilden, Robyn C., Katie Huffling, and Barbara Sattler. "Pesticides and health risks." *Journal of Obstetric, Gynecologic, and Neonatal Nursing: JOGNN* 39, no. 1 (2010): 103–110.

Hao, Shuang, Zhiqian Jia, Jianping Wen, Suoding Li, Wenjuan Peng, Renyao Huang, and Xin Xu. "Progress in adsorptive membranes for separation–A review." *Separation and Purification Technology* 255 (2021): 117772.

Heitner-Wirguin, Carla. "Recent advances in perfluorinated ionomer membranes: Structure, properties and applications." *Journal of Membrane Science* 120, no. 1 (1996): 1–33.

Huang, Dan-Lian, Rong-Zhong Wang, Yun-Guo Liu, Guang-Ming Zeng, Cui Lai, Piao Xu, Bing-An Lu, Juan-Juan Xu, Cong Wang, and Chao Huang. "Application of molecularly imprinted polymers in wastewater treatment: A review." *Environmental Science and Pollution Research International* 22, no. 2 (2015): 963–977.

Huang, Zheng-Qing, and Zheng-Fa Cheng. "Recent advances in adsorptive membranes for removal of harmful cations." *Journal of Applied Polymer Science* 137, no. 13 (2020): 48579.

Judd, Simon. *The MBR Book: Principles and Applications of Membrane Bioreactors for Water and Wastewater Treatment.* Elsevier, 2010.

Khataee, Alireza, Tannaz Sadeghi Rad, Sahand Nikzat, Aydin Hassani, Muhammed Hasan Aslan, Mehmet Kobya, and Erhan Demirbaş. "Fabrication of NiFe layered double hydroxide/reduced graphene oxide (NiFe-LDH/rGO) nanocomposite with enhanced sonophotocatalytic activity for the degradation of moxifloxacin." *Chemical Engineering Journal* 375 (2019): 122102.

Kıranşan, Murat, Alireza Khataee, Semra Karaca, and Mohsen Sheydaei. "Artificial neural network modeling of photocatalytic removal of a disperse dye using synthesized of ZnO nanoparticles on montmorillonite." *Spectrochimica Acta. Part A: Molecular and Biomolecular Spectroscopy* 140 (2015): 465–473.

Koe, Weng Shin, Jing Wen Lee, Woon Chan Chong, Yean Ling Pang, and Lan Ching Sim. "An overview of photocatalytic degradation: Photocatalysts, mechanisms, and development of photocatalytic membrane." *Environmental Science and Pollution Research International* 27, no. 3 (2020): 2522–2565.

Le-Clech, Pierre, Vicki Chen, and Tony A. G. Fane. "Fouling in membrane bioreactors used in wastewater treatment." *Journal of Membrane Science* 284, no. 1–2 (2006): 17–53.

Lee, Seul-Yi, and Soo-Jin Park. "TiO_2 photocatalyst for water treatment applications." *Journal of Industrial and Engineering Chemistry* 19, no. 6 (2013): 1761–1769.

Lhomme, L., S. Brosillon, and D. Wolbert. "Photocatalytic degradation of pesticides in pure water and a commercial agricultural solution on TiO_2 coated media." *Chemosphere* 70, no. 3 (2008): 381–386.

Li, Chengcheng, Corinne Cabassud, Bernard Reboul, and Christelle Guigui. "Effects of pharmaceutical micropollutants on the membrane fouling of a submerged MBR treating municipal wastewater: Case of continuous pollution by carbamazepine." *Water Research* 69 (2015): 183–194.

Li, Norman N., Anthony G. Fane, W. S. Winston Ho, and Takeshi Matsuura, eds. *Advanced Membrane Technology and Applications.* John Wiley & Sons, 2011.

Liang, Ze, Asem Mahmoud Abdelshafy, Zisheng Luo, Tarun Belwal, Xingyu Lin, Yanqun Xu, Lei Wang et al. "Occurrence, detection, and dissipation of pesticide residue in plant-derived foodstuff: A state-of-the-art review." *Food Chemistry* 384 (2022) 132494.

Litchfield, Sebastian G., Kai G. Schulz, and Brendan P. Kelaher. "The influence of plastic pollution and ocean change on detrital decomposition." *Marine Pollution Bulletin* 158 (2020): 111354.

Liu, Weiyi, Jinlan Zhang, Hang Liu, Xiaonan Guo, Xiyue Zhang, Xiaolong Yao, Zhiguo Cao, and Tingting Zhang. "A review of the removal of microplastics in global wastewater treatment plants: Characteristics and mechanisms." *Environment International* 146 (2021): 106277.

Lourthuraj, A. Amala, Mohammad Rafe Hatshan, and Dina S. Hussein. "Biocatalytic degradation of organophosphate pesticide from the wastewater and hydrolytic enzyme properties of consortium isolated from the pesticide contaminated water." *Environmental Research* 205 (2022): 112553.

Mandal, Mrinal Kanti, Manisha Sharma, Shailesh Pandey, and Kashyap Kumar Dubey. "Membrane technologies for the treatment of pharmaceutical industry wastewater." In: *Water and Wastewater Treatment Technologies*, pp. 103–116. Springer, Singapore, 2019.

Mansoori, Sepideh, Reza Davarnejad, Takeshi Matsuura, and Ahmad Fauzi Ismail. "Membranes based on non-synthetic (natural) polymers for wastewater treatment." *Polymer Testing* 84 (2020): 106381.

Miege, Cecile, J. M. Choubert, L. Ribeiro, M. Eusèbe, and Marina Coquery. "Fate of pharmaceuticals and personal care products in wastewater treatment plants–conception of a database and first results." *Environmental Pollution* 157, no. 5 (2009): 1721–1726.

Milić, Nataša, Maja Milanović, Nevena Grujić Letić, Maja Turk Sekulić, Jelena Radonić, Ivana Mihajlović, and Mirjana Vojinović Miloradov. "Occurrence of antibiotics as emerging contaminant substances in aquatic environment." *International Journal of Environmental Health Research* 23, no. 4 (2013): 296–310.

Molinari, Raffaele, Leonardo Palmisano, Enrico Drioli, and Mario Schiavello. "Studies on various reactor configurations for coupling photocatalysis and membrane processes in water purification." *Journal of Membrane Science* 206, no. 1–2 (2002): 399–415.

Montes-Grajales, Diana, Mary Fennix-Agudelo, and Wendy Miranda-Castro. "Occurrence of personal care products as emerging chemicals of concern in water resources: A review." *Science of the Total Environment* 595 (2017): 601–614.

Mozia, Sylwia. "Photocatalytic membrane reactors (PMRs) in water and wastewater treatment: A review." *Separation and Purification Technology* 73, no. 2 (2010): 71–91.

Mukherjee, Raka, Prasenjit Bhunia, and Sirshendu De. "Impact of graphene oxide on removal of heavy metals using mixed matrix membrane." *Chemical Engineering Journal* 292 (2016): 284–297.

Nasrollahi, Nazanin, Leila Ghalamchi, Vahid Vatanpour, and Alireza Khataee. "Photocatalytic-membrane technology: A critical review for membrane fouling mitigation." *Journal of Industrial and Engineering Chemistry* 93 (2021): 101–116.

Nunes, Suzana Pereira, and Klaus-Viktor Peinemann. *Membrane Technology*. Wiley-vch, 2001.

Oancea, Petruta, and Tatiana Oncescu. "The photocatalytic degradation of dichlorvos under solar irradiation." *Journal of Photochemistry and Photobiology, Part A: Chemistry* 199, no. 1 (2008): 8–13.

Ojha, Anupama, Santosh Kumar Yaduvanshi, Satish Chnadra Pant, Vinay Lomash, and Nalini Srivastava. "Evaluation of DNA damage and cytotoxicity induced by three commonly used organophosphate pesticides individually and in mixture, in rat tissues." *Environmental Toxicology* 28, no. 10 (2013): 543–552.

Patz, Jonathan A., Thaddeus K. Graczyk, Nina Geller, and Amy Y. Vittor. "Effects of environmental change on emerging parasitic diseases." *International Journal for Parasitology* 30, no. 12–13 (2000): 1395–1405.

Qalyoubi, Liyan, Amani Al-Othman, and Sameer Al-Asheh. "Recent progress and challenges on adsorptive membranes for the removal of pollutants from wastewater. Part I: Fundamentals and classification of membranes." *Case Studies in Chemical and Environmental Engineering* 3 (2021): 100086.

Ramli, Noor Hafizah, Suzana Yusup, Benjamin Wei Bin Kueh, Puteri Sarah Diba Kamarulzaman, Noridah Osman, Mardyahwati Abd Rahim, Ramlan Aziz, Sulaiman Mokhtar, and Abu Bakar Ahmad. "Effectiveness of biopesticides in enhancing paddy growth for yield improvement." *Sustainable Chemistry and Pharmacy* 7 (2018): 1–8.

Rathi, B. Senthil, P. Senthil Kumar, and Pau-Loke Show. "A review on effective removal of emerging contaminants from aquatic systems: Current trends and scope for further research." *Journal of Hazardous Materials* 409 (2021): 124413.

Ricky, R., and S. Shanthakumar. "Phycoremediation integrated approach for the removal of pharmaceuticals and personal care products from wastewater–A review." *Journal of Environmental Management* 302, no. A (2022): 113998.

Senthil Rathi, B., P. Senthil Kumar, and Pau-Loke Show. "A review on effective removal of emerging contaminants from aquatic systems: Current trends and scope for further research." *Journal of Hazardous Materials* 409 (2020): 124413.

Sharma, M. V., V. Phanikrishna, Durga Kumari, and M. Subrahmanyam. "TiO_2 supported over SBA-15: An efficient photocatalyst for the pesticide degradation using solar light." *Chemosphere* 73, no. 9 (2008): 1562–1569.

Shi, Yahui, Jinhui Huang, Guangming Zeng, Wenjian Cheng, and Jianglin Hu. "Photocatalytic membrane in water purification: Is it stepping closer to be driven by visible light?" *Journal of Membrane Science* 584 (2019): 364–392.

Silvestri, D., N. Barbani, C. Cristallini, Paolo Giusti, and G. Ciardelli. "Molecularly imprinted membranes for an improved recognition of biomolecules in aqueous medium." *Journal of Membrane Science* 282, no. 1–2 (2006): 284–295.

Sobiech, Monika, and Piotr Luliński. "Imprinted polymeric nanoparticles as nanodevices, biosensors and biolabels." In: *Nanostructures for the Engineering of Cells, Tissues and Organs*, pp. 331–374. William Andrew Publishing, 2018.

Taheran, Mehrdad, Mitra Naghdi, Satinder K. Brar, Mausam Verma, and Rao Y. Surampalli. "Emerging contaminants: Here today, there tomorrow!" *Environmental Nanotechnology, Monitoring and Management* 10 (2018): 122–126.

Tong, Hua, Shuxin Ouyang, Yingpu Bi, Naoto Umezawa, Mitsutake Oshikiri, and Jinhua Ye. "Nano-photocatalytic materials: Possibilities and challenges." *Advanced Materials* 24, no. 2 (2012): 229–251.

Tran, Ngoc Han, Martin Reinhard, and Karina Yew-Hoong Gin. "Occurrence and fate of emerging contaminants in municipal wastewater treatment plants from different geographical regions-a review." *Water Research* 133 (2018): 182–207.

Trotta, Francesco, Enrico Drioli, Claudio Baggiani, and Domenico Lacopo. "Molecular imprinted polymeric membrane for naringin recognition." *Journal of Membrane Science* 201, no. 1–2 (2002): 77–84.

Verlicchi, Paola, M. Al. Aukidy, and Elena Zambello. "Occurrence of pharmaceutical compounds in urban wastewater: Removal, mass load and environmental risk after a secondary treatment—A review." *Science of the Total Environment* 429 (2012): 123–155.

Verweij, Hendrik. "Inorganic membranes." *Current Opinion in Chemical Engineering* 1, no. 2 (2012): 156–162.

Vinh-Thang, Hoang, and Serge Kaliaguine. "Predictive models for mixed-matrix membrane performance: A review." *Chemical Reviews* 113, no. 7 (2013): 4980–5028.

Vo, Thi Sinh, Muhammad Mohsin Hossain, Hyung Mo Jeong, and Kyunghoon Kim. "Heavy metal removal applications using adsorptive membranes." *Nano Convergence* 7, no. 1 (2020): 1–26.

Wen, Qiang, Jiancheng Di, Yong Zhao, Yang Wang, Lei Jiang, and Jihong Yu. "Flexible inorganic nanofibrous membranes with hierarchical porosity for efficient water purification." *Chemical Science* 4, no. 12 (2013): 4378–4382.

Xu, Xiaojie, Lili Zhu, and Lirong Chen. "Separation and screening of compounds of biological origin using molecularly imprinted polymers." *Journal of Chromatography. Part B, Biomedical Sciences and Applications* 804, no. 1 (2004): 61–69.

Yoshikawa, Masakazu, Kalsang Tharpa, and Stefan-Ovidiu Dima. "Molecularly imprinted membranes: Past, present, and future." *Chemical Reviews* 116, no. 19 (2016): 11500–11528.

Zhang, Wenxiang, Luhui Ding, Jianquan Luo, Michel Y. Jaffrin, and Bing Tang. "Membrane fouling in photocatalytic membrane reactors (PMRs) for water and wastewater treatment: A critical review." *Chemical Engineering Journal* 302 (2016): 446–458.

Zheng, Xiang, Zhi-Peng Shen, Lei Shi, Rong Cheng, and Dong-Hai Yuan. "Photocatalytic membrane reactors (PMRs) in water treatment: Configurations and influencing factors." *Catalysts* 7, no. 8 (2017): 224.

Zou, Hanfa, Quanzhou Luo, and Dongmei Zhou. "Affinity membrane chromatography for the analysis and purification of proteins." *Journal of Biochemical and Biophysical Methods* 49, no. 1–3 (2001): 199–240.

9 Lassa Fever in Nigeria *Case Fatality Ratio, Social Consequences, and Prevention*

Sylvester Chibueze Izah, Adams Ovie Iyiola, Wisdom Richard Poyeri, and Kurotimipa Frank Ovuru

CONTENTS

9.1 Introduction 134
9.2 Origin and Epidemiology of Lassa Fever 135
9.2.1 Origin and Occurrence 135
9.2.2 Epidemiology of Lassa Fever 135
9.2.3 Signs and Symptoms of Lassa Fever 136
9.2.4 Mode of Transmission 136
9.2.5 Lassa Fever Vector 137
9.2.5.1 Mortality and Morbidity of Lassa Virus 138
9.2.6 Diagnosis, Treatment, and Prevention of Lassa Fever 138
9.2.6.1 Clinical Course 138
9.2.6.2 Diagnosis 138
9.2.6.3 Treatment 139
9.2.6.4 Prevention 139
9.2.7 Nigerian Public Health Response to Lassa Fever 141
9.3 Dynamics and Occurrence of Lassa Fever 141
9.3.1 Climatic Effects and Climate-Linked Dynamics of Lassa Fever. 141
9.3.2 Trends in Surveillance of Lassa Fever in Nigeria 142
9.4 Social Consequences of Lassa Fever 142
9.4.1 Stigma 142
9.4.1.1 Self-Stigma 143
9.4.1.2 Societal Stigma 143
9.4.2 Sensorineural Hearing Loss (SNHL) 143
9.4.3 Knowledge of Lassa Fever and Its Symptoms 144
9.4.4 Coping Strategies for Lassa Fever 144
9.5 Conclusion 144
References 145

DOI: 10.1201/9781003288732-9

9.1 INTRODUCTION

Mastomys natalensis is one of the most common agricultural pests in sections of sub-Saharan Africa. It is found in large numbers in various human-dominated land types, with reduced abundance in natural and wooded ecosystems compared with human-dominated land types. This animal host is native to Nigeria and the West African sub-region and serves as food to some populations across Nigeria. This mouse species' populations show substantial seasonal dynamics that vary among habitat types, likely connected to changes in food supply throughout time (Fichet-Calvet et al., 2007).

The multimammate rat (*Mastomys natalensis*) spread Lassa virus to humans. Hence, Lassa fever is a zoonotic disease and is widespread in West Africa, where it has caused significant health concerns. Lassa infection is due to an arenavirus that causes Lassa haemorrhagic fever.

Nigeria has, in recent times, periodically suffered from Lassa fever epidemics. The disease is reported to be endemic in Nigeria. The upsurge in reported virus cases in parts of Nigeria is worrisome and of great concern. Death from the disease occurs in approximately 15–20% of cases (Bajani et al., 1997). As a result of the high rate of occurrence, Lassa fever has become a significant issue not just in Nigeria but across the West African region. Some other countries regularly impacted by Lassa fever in the sub-region include Sierra Leone, Ghana, Benin, Guinea, Mali, and Liberia. This concern has been raised several times on the sidelines of meetings of the Economic Community of West African States (ECOWAS) in order to prevent its spread and curtail its outbreak.

The Lassa virus enters the host cell through the alpha-dystroglycan (alpha-DG) cell-surface receptor (Oppliger et al., 2016). The alpha-dystroglycan is a multifunctional extracellular matrix protein receptor. The prototypic arenavirus lymphocytic choriomeningitis virus shares this receptor. The large proteins, a category of glycosyltransferases, modify alpha-dystroglycan with a particular sugar modification for receptor binding. Many people infected with the virus may not have symptoms right away, and in some cases, symptoms appear gradually. When symptoms appear, they include flu-like symptoms such as fever, general weakness, cough, sore throat, headache, and gastrointestinal indications. Vascular permeability is one of the haemorrhagic symptoms (Yun and Walker, 2012).

The incubation period for the Lassa virus ranges from 2 to 21 days, and transmission is mostly by contact with stored grains or food contaminated with the faeces or urine of rodents in households. The causative agent of the disease is shed in the rodent's excreta (urine and faeces) and can be aerosolised. Therefore, any person suspected of having contracted Lassa fever should be immediately quarantined in an isolation facility. Body fluids and faeces of such person(s) infected with the Lassa virus should be appropriately disposed of while treatment is administered to avoid secondary transmission. Persons living in rural settlements with poor sanitation conditions and habits where *Mastomys* are predominant are at higher risk of contracting the disease when compared with those in urban settlements with better sanitary conditions and habits. This factor has greatly enhanced the spread of the disease across Nigeria because of poor sanitation and hygiene practices, with higher numbers in the north, where the virus was first discovered. Therefore, the Lassa fever disease is a public health concern that presently constitutes an infectious menace in Nigeria and parts of the African continent; hence, efforts must be deliberately made to curb it without delay whenever an incident is reported. There is also a need for continuous awareness creation and sensitisation of the general public, especially in high-risk environments.

9.2 ORIGIN AND EPIDEMIOLOGY OF LASSA FEVER

9.2.1 Origin and Occurrence

Lassa fever is a viral illness that originates from animals. It is predominant in West African countries like Sierra Leone, Guinea, Liberia, and Nigeria. Countries around the West African region are vulnerable to this virus because the animal vector of this disease, the multimammate rat (*Mastomys natalensis*), is well distributed around these regions. Lassa fever virus belongs to the arenavirus family and was identified in 1969 after its first description in the 1950s. The illness was given the name after a Nigerian town called 'Lassa,' where the first case of this illness occurred, leading to the death of two missionaries (Dan-Nwafor et al., 2019; Asogun et al., 2012). It has been estimated that approximately 5,000 deaths occur yearly from this illness, with an infection rate of 100,000 to 300,000. The disease has been reported to have serious effects in some areas of Liberia and Sierra Leone, with many cases of hospitalisation, as high as 10–16% of the total populace (NCDC, 2020; Centers for Disease Control and Prevention, 2019; Bausch et al., 2001).

In Nigeria, as of week 8 in 2022, the cumulative suspected cases, confirmed cases, probable cases, deaths confirmed, case fatality ratio, affected states, and affected local government areas (LGAs) were 2,433, 540, 20, 98, 18.1%, 21, and 79, respectively, whereas in week 8 of 2021, the corresponding numbers were 959, 136, 2, 31, 22.8%, 11, and 40, respectively (NCDC, 2022). The fever has a peak period of occurrence in the dry season (December–April), and it is endemic to Nigeria. The reduced capacity in testing and surveillance has led to an increased epidemic occurrence compared with previous years.

9.2.2 Epidemiology of Lassa Fever

The fever is a systemic viral infection caused by a single-stranded RNA virus (Lowe et al., 2016; Healing and Gopal, 2001; Johnson et al., 1987). Fulminant viraemia is the main feature of the illness, and it can impair or delay cellular immunity (Cheng and Cosgriff, 2000). It has been reported that the prevalence of human antibodies to the virus is 8–52% in Sierra Leone (McCormick et al., 1987), 4–55% in Guinea (Lukashevich et al., 1993), and 21% in Nigeria (Tomori et al., 1988). In addition, seropositivity of human infection has been reported in countries like the Central African Republic, Mali, Congo DRC, and Senegal. Cases have also been reported in travellers who returned to Britain, Germany, and the

Netherlands. The years when Lassa fever cases were first confirmed in African countries include 2011 in Ghana and the DRC, and 2014 in the Benin Republic. Endemic countries for Lassa fever include Guinea, with Kindia, Faranah, and Nzerekore regions having most outbreaks occurring between May and December 2021; Liberia, with Lofa, Bong, and Nimba being areas of intense transmission and an outbreak occurring in the UN mission in Kakata Margibi County in 2014; Nigeria, with different parts affected by peaks occurring in the dry season between December and February,; and Sierra Leone, in Kenema and Kailahun districts, with recent evidence of changes in geographical spread (UK Health Security Agency, 2014).

9.2.3 Signs and Symptoms of Lassa Fever

Symptoms appear between 1 and 3 weeks after contracting the virus. Mild symptoms such as weakness, fever, and headache are generally observed in most infected patients (about 80%). In severe cases, symptoms such as haemorrhaging, continuous vomiting, swellings on the face, and chest, abdominal, and back pains are observed. Neurological problems such as tremors and hearing loss have also been reported. Death usually occurs 2 weeks after the onset of disease because the body organs will have been seriously damaged. Deafness of various degrees is the most common complication arising from the virus. Eventually, it results in permanent deafness in both mild and extreme cases of viral infection.

The diagnosis of the fever is varied and non-specific, so it is difficult to diagnose the virus clinically. Therefore, about 15–20% of people who are hospitalised for Lassa illness die from it. Fatal cases are rampant in pregnant women in their third trimester of pregnancy, and 95% of such cases result in the abortion of fetuses (Amorosa et al., 2010).

9.2.4 Mode of Transmission

The multimammate rat (*Mastomys natalensis*) is the host of the virus. The rodent can spread the virus via urine once it is infected. Rodents of this species are prolific breeders and are abundant in the forests and savannahs of West, East, and Central Africa. These rodents are usually found in residential buildings and have the ability to populate areas where foods are stored in homes. This medium easily transfers the virus from rodents to humans (Figure 9.1).

The virus is transferred to humans through two major processes:

- Inhalation
- Ingestion

Infections are spread when there is direct contact with materials infected by the urine or droppings of the rodents. These viruses are deposited and can be contacted by touching contaminated objects, by eating contaminated food, or via exposed cuts and sores on humans. This indicates that the virus can also be spread

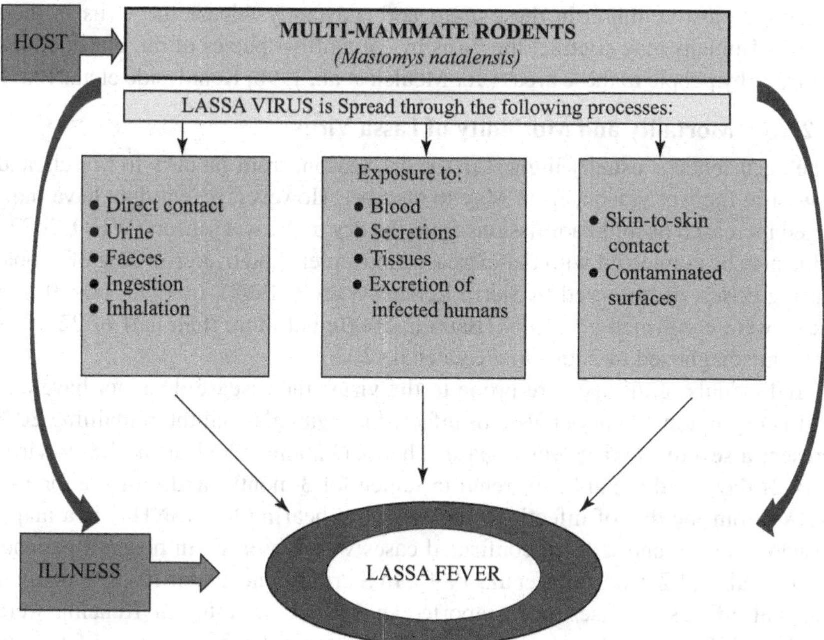

FIGURE 9.1 Mode of transmission of Lassa fever.

through sores and cuts rather than by ingesting contaminated food (Crowfort, 2002; Cummins et al., 1990).

Contact transmission of the virus is most common because rodents living around residential homes scavenge on improperly kept or leftover food. Contact with such items can cause disease transmission. In addition, the rodent may be consumed as food in some areas, thereby transferring the virus to humans despite the preparation method. The virus can also be spread through faecally contaminated air, especially when cleaning and sweeping rodent-infested areas.

Apart from spreading through rodents, person-to-person transmission can also occur when exposed to virus-contaminated blood or contaminated tissues, secretions, and excretions of infected individuals. Casual contact, such as skin-to-skin contact, can also spread the virus from person to person without exchanging bodily fluids. Therefore, wearing personal protective equipment (PPE) in health centres is vital because person-to-person transmission is predominant in these areas. Contaminated machines and equipment in health centres can also be a medium for virus spread (Centers for Disease Control and Prevention, 2019; Fichet-Calvet et al., 2014).

9.2.5 Lassa Fever Vector

M. natalensis is a host for the Lassa virus. These rodents breed frequently and are distributed throughout Central, West, and East Africa (Healing and Gopal, 2001).

They are most common in these areas and constantly release the virus in their faeces. Humans may contract the virus by eating this species of rat, considered a delicacy by people in these areas (Ter Meulen et al., 1996; Kennlyside et al., 1983).

9.2.5.1 Mortality and Morbidity of Lassa Virus

The occurrence is usually highest in the dry season, from January to March, and lowest in the wet season, from May to October. However, recent data have indicated increased hospital admissions from the dry to the wet season (WHO, 2022). This may be connected with the increased movement and overcrowding of people during crises, as observed in Sierra Leone (Wilson, 1995). In 1998, 60–70% of cases were confirmed clinically (Bausch, 2000), but more than half of 22 cases were misdiagnosed in 2000 (Ipadeola et al., 2020).

Individuals of all ages are prone to the virus; the disease does not have any distinct symptoms in about 80% of infected individuals, and the remaining 20% present a severe multisystem disease. The incubation period of the Lassa virus is 6–21 days, and it can be excreted in semen for 3 months and in urine for 3–9 weeks from the day of infection. Sensorineural hearing loss (SNHL) is a major disease feature, and 29% of confirmed cases were observed in hospital patients (Liao et al., 1992; Cummins et al., 1990). In Sierra Leone, about 10–16% of adult hospital admission cases were reported in 1987. Case rates in Kenema were between 12% and 23% from 1997 to 2002. Maternal deaths (29%) and fetal and neonatal loss (87%) were reported during pregnancy, and a 25% maternal death rate was reported in Sierra Leone. The virus also infected Peacekeepers in Sierra Leone (Ter Meulen et al., 2001). From July to September 2002, 11 admissions from the army and 10 from UN missions were reported, with 1 individual death from each group (Price et al., 1988).

9.2.6 Diagnosis, Treatment, and Prevention of Lassa Fever

9.2.6.1 Clinical Course

The signs and symptoms of the illness are similar to those of malaria and Ebola. The clinical stages of the disease are presented in Figure 9.2 (McCarthy, 2002). It is challenging to diagnose clinically, but cases of patients with body temperature of ≥38 °C and not showing signs of response to antimalarials and antibiotics are suspected cases of Lassa illness. The clinical signs are fever, pain, pharyngitis, proteinuria, fever, vomiting, and sore throat (McCormick et al., 1987). The complications of the illness include bleeding in the mucosal membranes (17%), pleural effusion (3%), sensorineural hearing deficit (4%), and pericardial effusion (2%) (Johnson et al., 1987; McCormick et al., 1987).

9.2.6.2 Diagnosis

After the symptoms are observed, the infection can be diagnosed using the enzyme-linked immunosorbent serologic assay (ELISA). This process can detect IgM and IgG antibodies and the antigen of Lassa. At the early stage of Lassa fever, the reverse transcription-polymerase chain reaction (RT-PCR) is used for

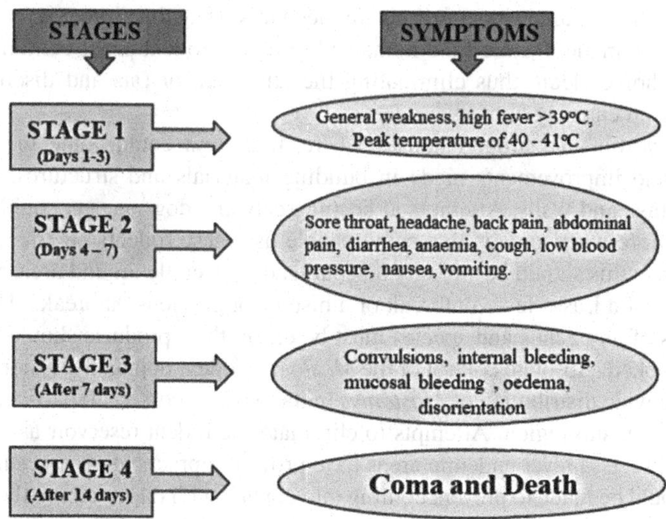

FIGURE 9.2 Clinical stages of Lassa illness.

diagnosis (Rottingen et al., 2017; Frame, 1992). The virus can be isolated and cultured for 7 to 10 days for investigation, but care must be taken. The laboratory must be free from contamination and have good practices. Post-mortem diagnosis can be carried out using immunohistochemistry practices on tissue specimens fixed with formalin (Demby et al., 1994).

9.2.6.3 Treatment

An antiviral drug called Ribavirin is used for treatment, and success rates have been observed. This drug is most effective when used during the early stages of the fever. Intensive care is also required for patients who must receive fluids to balance body electrolytes (Besen et al., 2015). Ribavirin is very effective when administered intravenously rather than orally, and the death rate can be reduced by 90% if treatment is started within the first 6 days of illness. Issues such as oedema, hypotension, fluid replacement or blood transfusion should be monitored carefully (Johnson et al., 1987).

9.2.6.4 Prevention

Given the problems connected with controlling the *Mastomys* rat population, the vector that causes Lassa fever presents one of the most serious public health concerns. This makes Lassa fever management difficult; nonetheless, measures aimed at keeping the animal host out of food supplies and residences, and appropriate human hygiene maintenance, are critical. In addition, the major mechanism by which the virus spreads from its host to humans can be avoided by taking steps to limit *Mastomys* contact with humans in areas where the disease is spreading.

Promoting good community hygiene to deter rodents from entering homes, encouraging effective personal hygiene, and disposing of garbage far from residential homes are critical preventive mechanisms against Lassa fever. Efforts must also be made to store food items and grains in rodent-proof containers and keep the home clean, thus eliminating the attraction of rats and discouraging rodents from entering homes.

Holes within and around houses where *Mastomys* could come in must be blocked and improvements made in building materials and structures, particularly ceilings and walls. Attempts at keeping cats and dogs as pets could also be helpful. More worrisome is that some people use these rodents (*Mastomys*) as a food source; this should be strongly discouraged, especially around areas with the likelihood of a Lassa fever outbreak or a history of previous outbreaks. However, if rodents of any genus and species must be eaten, their products should be thoroughly cooked. Absolute control of the *Mastomys* rodent population is not feasible due to the wide distribution of *Mastomys* in the African continent, particularly the West African sub-region. Attempts to eliminate the rodent reservoir as a control measure in Lassa fever endemic areas have proven impractical. As a result, every effort should be made to prevent coming into contact with rats or eating their meat. If rats must be handled, gloves and other protective clothes should be worn.

As a control measure, persons suspected of having contracted the virus should be quarantined in special isolation centres, and upon confirmation of the presence of the virus, efforts should be put in place to ensure faeces and body fluids of infected persons are adequately disposed of. Family members of such sick persons should be educated appropriately to avoid contact with blood and body fluids while caring for their sick relatives. The same applies to medical personnel who provide care to ill patients. This is because continued transmission of Lassa fever through person-to-person contact could occur when caring for people with the disease. To prevent this, considerable efforts and preventive steps must be taken to avoid contact with patient secretions. This can be accomplished by wearing appropriate PPE, such as masks, gloves, gowns, and goggles; infection control procedures, such as complete equipment sterilisation and separating infected patients from unprotected individuals until the disease has run its course, should be implemented. The patient may continue to excrete the virus in urine or sperm for weeks after recovery; thus, body fluids should be checked for infectivity before the patient is released. Meanwhile, a counselling programme emphasising the disinfection of toilets before use and sexual partner protection should be implemented. People who work in medical laboratories where samples are taken from humans and animals to examine for Lassa virus infection are also at risk; hence, such samples should only be handled by trained personnel and processed under the strictest biological containment settings possible.

In a healthcare setting, standard precautions should be used with all patients. This comprises a set of standard procedures that everyone must use, regardless of their illness status. Workers should always use conventional infection prevention and control (IPC) practices when caring for patients. Respiratory hygiene, using PPE (to prevent splashing or other contacts with infectious materials), and proper injection and burial methods should all be part of these safeguards.

Handwashing techniques and the safe handling and disposal of used needles and syringes in the hospital environment are critical to preventing and controlling

Lassa fever outbreaks not just in Nigeria but also around the world. Handwashing with soap and water removes microorganisms from the skin and hands, providing some protection against transmission of the virus and other diseases. As part of its guidelines for the management of Lassa fever cases in Nigeria, the Nigeria Centre for Disease Control (NCDC) recommends that hand hygiene be performed before and after any direct contact between a healthcare worker and a patient, and contact between patients, in the following scenarios, regardless of whether gloves are worn or not: upon entry into the isolation area, and before putting on PPE (NCDC, 2018).

9.2.7 Nigerian Public Health Response to Lassa Fever

- Coordination

The NCDC launched a National Emergency Operations alert for optimal monitoring, coordination, and a multi-disciplinary approach to the virus. The National Rapid Response Teams (NRRT) were deployed to states with severe cases

- Case Management and Infection Prevention and Control (IPC)

IPC guidelines were circulated, and training was organised for healthcare and public health workers

- Surveillance

The monitoring and surveillance of the virus are currently ongoing, and data are used for simulation studies and other responsive plans

- Clinical Management

Confirmed cases are treated, and medical facilities for treatment are being distributed around the country's states

- Laboratory Capacity

The national Lassa fever laboratories perform optimal analysis and processing of samples in the country for rapid response (WHO, 2022, Bausch et al., 2000)

9.3 Dynamics and Occurrence of Lassa Fever

9.3.1 Climatic Effects and Climate-Linked Dynamics of Lassa Fever

Understanding the dynamics based on climate and geography will go a long way towards informing Lassa fever diagnosis, prevention, and control. The spatio-temporal climatic incidences can be modelled to account for the disease's baseline information and expansion in surveillance and seasonality. Climate variability is associated with the seasonality of Lassa fever in timing and amplitude. A study during the outbreak in 2018 illustrated a high, climatic-driven risk in the southern part of Nigeria (Ehichioya et al., 2019). The seasonal Lassa fever risk was also associated with rainfall distribution and decline in vegetation. The study concluded that vegetation and rainfall dynamics affect Lassa fever incidence in Nigeria. Agricultural and food storage practices can influence the variation in rodent numbers and the Lassa fever virus in humans (Gibb et al., 2017; Massawe et al., 2007).

9.3.2 Trends in Surveillance of Lassa Fever in Nigeria

The weekly epidemiological reports of Lassa fever cases compiled by the NCDC were collected from 774 LGAs between 2012 and 2019. About 161 LGAs reported cases in 32 out of the 36 states in Nigeria, and there were 276 confirmed cases. Most reported cases were from 3 (Ondo, Edo and Ebonyi states) out of 36 states in Nigeria, while the others had low case reports. Seasonality was experienced in all areas of reported cases except in 2014–2015, when reported cases coincided with the Ebola outbreak. Lassa fever cases usually peak in the dry season in January as confirmed from data in Nigeria (Akpede et al., 2019; Asogun et al., 2012) and Sierra Leone (Shaffer et al., 2014). Secondary peak periods were also reported in March, with fewer cases reported throughout the year (Akpede et al., 2018). During the monitoring period in Nigeria from 2012 to 2019, NCDC was directly involved in the surveillance of Lassa fever by establishing a dedicated NCDC Technical Working Group in 2016. This led three diagnostic laboratories to diagnose the virus in 2017–2019 (Ilori et al., 2019). In addition, reporting systems with mobile phones were deployed in 18 states in 2017 (Siddle et al., 2018; NCDC, 2016). These measures flattened the virus curve between 2018 and 2019.

Most of the reported Lassa cases were from Esan Central in Edo State from 2012 to 2015, and this area is where the longest-serving Lassa fever diagnostic laboratory and treatment centre in Nigeria is located. The laboratory is domiciled in Irrua Specialist Teaching Hospital (ISTH) (Akpede et al., 2019; Asogun et al., 2012). The Lassa fever cases were observed to increase in 2016, but a decline occurred in cases from Esan Central and the surrounding local governments.

9.4 SOCIAL CONSEQUENCES OF LASSA FEVER

9.4.1 Stigma

The stigma resulting from Lassa fever infection can affect patients by destroying the psychosocial welfare of vulnerable people. They are often rejected by friends and family who are not willing to care for them in their state of illness (Olayemi et al., 2016). Stigmatisation is a serious issue that greatly affects disadvantaged people when healthcare is required. Addressing this issue requires interventions to tackle the lived experiences of infected people. An occurrence was observed in the 2018 outbreak of Lassa in which health workers kept a distance from infected patients to avoid being infected (Olayemi et al., 2018). Some who made contact were asked to isolate themselves by staying indoors in order not to spread the infection. This stigmatisation is widespread among healthcare workers who treat the disease. Some patients who have recovered from the disease also experience some form of stigmatisation from friends and families (Lo Iacono et al., 2015).

The following policies may be recommended to reduce the occurrence of stigmatisation.

- Provision of support by the government and friends for areas where Lassa fever and hearing loss are endemic
- Provision of information in ways that infected patients can understand. In this way, the information disseminated will be accurate, reducing discrimination (Zhao et al., 2020; Sogoba et al., 2016)

9.4.1.1 Self-Stigma

Infected people can experience this form of stigma at various levels, and some drivers are:

- Rejection or denial by people
- Fear of re-infection and infecting others around

In a study by Idigbe et al. (2020) in Ondo State on Lassa fever occurrence, most respondents denied the result when they were diagnosed with Lassa fever. The major question asked was the fear of infecting others, especially their close relatives. Over 50% of the diagnosed patients asked if there was a cure for the disease and about the fear of being re-infected if treated. A lot of the respondents also expressed fear of disclosing their health status to their relatives (Massawe et al., 2007).

9.4.1.2 Societal Stigma

Idigbe et al. (2020) used the following drivers to assess the societal stigma:

- Alienation
- Response of community to Lassa fever
- Perception of the society of Lassa fever

The study noted that many people perceived the disease as contagious and stayed away from the infected persons and people with whom they may have interacted. To reduce this, programmes and workshops must educate people about the disease. This will significantly reduce social discrimination (Asogun et al., 2012; Ehichioya et al., 2010; Fisher-Hosh et al., 1995).

9.4.2 Sensorineural Hearing Loss (SNHL)

Loss of hearing is a major sign of Lassa illness, and in 1990, the relationship with sudden-onset SNHL was clinically confirmed. SNHF affects one in every three infected individuals and can become a social burden (Mayrhuber et al., 2017). The quality of life and interaction is reduced in infected individuals with hearing loss, costing as much as 43 million dollars per year (Akpede et al., 2019; Akpede et al., 2018; Ballester et al., 2016). Also, the lack of samples for autopsy has limited the development of vaccines and treatment measures for the disease. Therefore, a model was created, mimicking all the symptoms of SNHL caused by Lassa fever. The data derived from this model supported the mechanism of immune-mediated injuries that usually cause SNHL scenarios in patients with Lassa fever (NCDC, 2012; Tomori et al., 1988). Furthermore, research is required to identify the epidemiology of SNHL cases induced by Lassa fever (Mateer et al., 2018).

9.4.3 Knowledge of Lassa Fever and Its Symptoms

Information dissemination and training about the prevention, causes, and treatment of Lassa fever are essential so that can handle the cases of illness better. Proper hygiene and environmental sanitation will also be encouraged to reduce the occurrence of the illness (Inegbenebor et al., 2010). Healthcare workers and officers will also stimulate precautionary measures via this medium by aligning with the culture, traditional practices, and customs (Ogbu et al., 2007; Omilabi et al., 2005).

9.4.4 Coping Strategies for Lassa Fever

All respondents said that coping with the medicines, being labelled a 'Lassa Fever Person,' and being reintegrated into society following treatment were challenging aspects of their diagnosis and treatment that they did not want to revisit (Akhmetzhanov et al., 2019). As a result, they feel that establishing counselling centres and support lines nearby will help eliminate stigma and create opportunities and platforms for them to discuss ways and tactics to cope with Lassa fever (Frame et al., 1970). It will also give the families who help with treatment the skills they need to care for Lassa fever survivors. Asogun et al. (2014), investigating 'Dealing with the Unseen: Fear and Stigma' in Irrua, Edo State, found that self and societal stigma exist. This corroborates another study by Mayrhuber et al. (2017) on Ebola survivors: 'We are Survivors and not a Virus: Content analysis of media reporting on Ebola survivors in Liberia' (Anderson et al., 2015; VHFC, 2013; McCormick, 1987).

9.5 CONCLUSION

Lassa fever is a severe viral infection that affects people in West Africa. The disease is caused by a single-stranded RNA virus that belongs to the Arenaviridae virus family. The virus is zoonotic because it is vectored by a multimammate rat (*Mastomys natalensis*). Nigeria is one of the major nations or countries where Lassa fever is endemic. The infection rate of the disease in West Africa is between

100,000 and 300,000, with about 5,000 deaths annually. However, in Nigeria (Week 8; 21–27 February 2022), the case fatality ratio is 18.1%, which is lower than 22.8% reported in the same period in 2021. Therefore, a major tool for preventing and controlling Lassa fever in Nigeria will be to constantly create awareness about the virus and continuously educate the people in high-risk areas about ways to reduce rodent populations in their homes. The good news is that there are current research efforts to develop a vaccine for Lassa fever.

REFERENCES

Akhmetzhanov, A.R., Asai, Y. and Nishiura, H., 2019. Quantifying the seasonal drivers of transmission for Lassa fever in Nigeria. *Philosophical Transactions of the Royal Society Series B*, *374*(1775), p.20180268.

Akpede, G.O., Asogun, D.A., Okogbenin, S.A., Dawodu, S.O., Momoh, M.O., Dongo, A.E., Ike, C., Tobin, E., Akpede, N., Ogbaini-Emovon, E. and Adewale, A.E., 2019. Caseload and case fatality of Lassa fever in Nigeria, 2001–2018: A specialist center's experience and its implications. *Frontiers in Public Health*, *7*, p.170.

Akpede, G.O., Asogun, D.A., Okogbenin, S.A. and Okokhere, P.O., 2018. Lassa fever outbreaks in Nigeria. *Expert Review of Anti-Infective Therapy*, *16*(9), pp.663–666.

Amorosa, V., MacNeil, A., McConnell, R., Patel, A., Dillon, K.E., Hamilton, K., Erickson, B.R., Campbell, S., Knust, B., Cannon, D. and Miller, D., 2010. Imported Lassa fever, Pennsylvania, USA, 2010. *Emerging Infectious Diseases*, *16*(10), p.1598.

Andersen, K., Jesse Shapiro, B., Matranga, C., Sealfon, R., Lin, A., Moses, L., Folarin, O., Goba, A., Odia, I., Ehiane, P. and Momoh, M., 2015. Clinical sequencing uncovers origins and evolution of Lassa virus. *Cell*, *162*(4), pp.738–750.

Asogun, D., Tobin, E.A., Gunther, S., Happi, C. and Ikponwosa, O., 2014. Dealing with the unseen: Ffear and stigma in Lassa fever. *International Journal of Infectious Diseases*, *21*, p.221.

Asogun, D.A., Adomeh, D.I., Ehimuan, J., Odia, I., Hass, M., Gabriel, M., Ölschläger, S., Becker-Ziaja, B., Folarin, O., Phelan, E. and Ehiane, P.E., 2012. Molecular diagnostics for Lassa fever at Irrua specialist teaching hospital, Nigeria: Lessons learnt from two years of laboratory operation. *PLOS Neglected Tropical Diseases*, *6*, p. e1839. https://doi.org/10.1371/journal.pntd.0001839.

Bajani, M.D., Tomori, O., Rollin, P.E., Harry, T.O., Bukbuk, N.D., Wilson, L., Childs, J.E., Peters, C.J. and Ksiazek, T.G., 1997. A survey for antibodies to Lassa virus among health workers in Nigeria. *Transactions of the Royal Society of Tropical Medicine and Hygiene*, *91*(4), pp.379–381.

Ballester, J., Lowe, R., Diggle, P.J. and Rodó, X., 2016. Seasonal forecasting and health impact models: Challenges and opportunities. *Annals of the New York Academy of Sciences*, *1382*(1), pp.8–20.

Bausch, D.G., 2000. *Lassa Fever in Sierra Leone*. London: Merlin.

Bausch, D.G., Demby, A.H., Coulibaly, M., Kanu, J., Goba, A., Bah, A., Conde, N., Wurtzel, H.L., Cavallaro, K.F., Lloyd, E. and Baldet, F.B., 2001. Lassa fever in Guinea: I. Epidemiology of human disease and clinical observations. *Vector Borne and Zoonotic Diseases*, *1*(4), pp.269–281.

Bausch, D.G., Rollin, P.E., Demby, A.H., Coulibaly, M., Kanu, J., Conteh, A.S., Wagoner, K.D., McMullan, L.K., Bowen, M.D., Peters, C.J. and Ksiazek, T.G., 2000. Diagnosis and clinical virology of Lassa fever as evaluated by enzyme-linked immunosorbent assay, indirect fluorescent-antibody test, and virus isolation. *Journal of Clinical Microbiology*, *38*(7), pp.2670–2677.

Beesen, B.A.M.P., Gobatto, A.L.N., Merlo, L.M.G., Maciel, A.T. and Park, M., 2015. Fluid and electrolyte overload in critically ill patients: An overview. *World Journal of Critical Care Medicine*, *4*(2), pp.116–129. https://www.doi.org/10.5492/wjccm.v4.i2.116.

Centers for Disease Control and Prevention, 2019. Lassa fever. https://www.cdc.gov/vhf/lassa/.

Chen, J.P. and Cosgriff, T.M., 2000. Hemorrhagic fever virus-induced changes in hemostasis and vascular biology. *Blood Coagulation and Fibrinolysis*, *11*(5), pp.461–483.

Crowcroft, N., 2002. Management of Lassa fever in European countries. *Eurosurveillance*, *7*(3), pp.50–52.

Cummins, D., McCormick, J.B., Bennett, D., Samba, J.A., Farrar, B., Machin, S.J. and Fisher-Hoch, S.P., 1990. Acute sensorineural deafness in Lassa fever. *JAMA*, *264*(16), pp.2093–2096.

Dan-Nwafor, C.C., Furuse, Y., Ilori, E.A., Ipadeola, O., Akabike, K.O., Ahumibe, A., Ukponu, W., Bakare, L., Okwor, T.J., Joseph, G. and Mba, N.G., 2019. Measures to control protracted large Lassa fever outbreak in Nigeria, 1 January to 28 April 2019. *Eurosurveillance*, 24(20), p.1900272.

Demby, A.H., Chamberlain, J., Brown, D.W. and Clegg, C.S., 1994. Early diagnosis of Lassa fever by reverse transcription-PCR. *Journal of Clinical Microbiology*, *32*(12), pp.2898–2903.

Ehichioya, D.U., Dellicour, S., Pahlmann, M., Rieger, T., Oestereich, L., Becker-Ziaja, B., Cadar, D., Ighodalo, Y., Olokor, T., Omomoh, E. and Oyakhilome, J., 2019. Phylogeography of Lassa virus in Nigeria. *Journal of Virology*, *93*(21), p.e00929-19.

Ehichioya, D.U., Hass, M., Ölschläger, S., Becker-Ziaja, B., Chukwu, C.O.O., Coker, J., Nasidi, A., Ogugua, O.O., Günther, S. and Omilabu, S.A., 2010. Lassa fever, Nigeria, 2005–2008. *Emerging Infectious Diseases*, *16*(6), pp.1040–1041.

Fichet-Calvet, E., Becker-Ziaja, B., Koivogui, L. and Günther, S., 2014. Lassa serology in natural populations of rodents and horizontal transmission. *Vector Borne and Zoonotic Diseases*, *14*(9), pp.665–674.

Fichet-Calvet, E., Lecompte, E., Koivogui, L., Soropogui, B., Doré, A., Kourouma, F., Sylla, O., Daffis, S., Koulémou, K. and Meulen, J.T., 2007. Fluctuation of abundance and Lassa virus prevalence in Mastomys natalensis in Guinea, West Africa. *Vector Borne and Zoonotic Diseases*, *7*(2), pp.119–128.

Fisher-Hoch, S.P., Tomori, O., Nasidi, A., Perez-Oronoz, G.I., Fakile, Y., Hutwagner, L. and McCormick, J.B., 1995. Review of cases of nosocomial Lassa fever in Nigeria: The high price of poor medical practice. *BMJ: British Medical Journal*, *311*(7009), pp.857–859.

Frame, J.D., 1992. The story of Lassa fever. Part I: Discovering the disease. *New York State Journal of Medicine*, *92*(5), pp.199–202.

Frame, J.D., Baldwin Jr, J.M., Gocke, D.J. and Troup, J.M., 1970. Lassa fever, a new virus disease of man from West Africa. I. Clinical description and pathological findings. *The American Journal of Tropical Medicine and Hygiene*, *19*(4), pp.670–676.

Gibb, R., Moses, L.M., Redding, D.W. and Jones, K.E., 2017. Understanding the cryptic nature of Lassa fever in West Africa. *Pathogens and Global Health*, *111*(6), pp.276–288.

Healing, T. and Gopal, R., 2001. *Report on an Assessment Visit to Sierra Leone, April 12th–30th 2001*. London: Merlin.

Idigbe, I.E., Salu, O.B., Amoo, O.S., Musa, A.Z., Shaibu, J.O., Abejegah, C., Ayodeji, O.O., Ezechi, O.C., Omilabu, S.A., Audu, R.A. and Salako, B.L., 2020. Dealing with stigma and its impact on Lassa-fever survivors in Ondo state. *Trends in Research*, *3*(2). https://doi.org/10.15761/TR.1000158.

Ilori, E.A., Frank, C., Dan-Nwafor, C.C., Ipadeola, O., Krings, A., Ukponu, W., Womi-Eteng, O.E., Adeyemo, A., Mutbam, S.K., Musa, E.O. and Lasuba, C.L., 2019. Increase in Lassa fever cases in Nigeria, January–March 2018. *Emerging Infectious Diseases*, *25*(5), pp.1026–1027.

Inegbenebor, U., Okosun, J. and Inegbenebor, J., 2010. Prevention of Lassa fever in Nigeria. *Transactions of the Royal Society of Tropical Medicine and Hygiene*, *104*(1), pp.51–54.

Ipadeola, O., Furuse, Y., Ilori, E.A., Dan-Nwafor, C.C., Akabike, K.O., Ahumibe, A., Ukponu, W., Bakare, L., Joseph, G., Saleh, M. and Muwanguzi, E.N., 2020. Epidemiology and case-control study of Lassa fever outbreak in Nigeria from 2018 to 2019. *Journal of Infection*, *80*(5), pp.578–606.

Johnson, K.M., McCormick, J.B., Webb, P.A., Smith, E.S., Elliott, L.H. and King, I.J., 1987. Clinical virology of Lassa fever in hospitalized patients. *Journal of Infectious Diseases*, *155*(3), pp.456–464.

Keenlyside, R.A., McCormick, J.B., Webb, P.A., Smith, E., Elliott, L. and Johnson, K.M., 1983. Case-control study of Mastomys natalensis and humans in Lassa virus-infected households in Sierra Leone. *The American Journal of Tropical Medicine and Hygiene*, *32*(4), pp.829–837.

Liao, B.S., Byl, F.M. and Adour, K.K., 1992. Audiometric comparison of Lassa fever hearing loss and idiopathic sudden hearing loss: Evidence for viral cause. *Otolaryngology. Otolaryngology–Head and Neck Surgery*, *106*(3), pp.226–229.

Lo Iacono, G., Cunningham, A.A., Fichet-Calvet, E., Garry, R.F., Grant, D.S., Khan, S.H., Leach, M., Moses, L.M., Schieffelin, J.S., Shaffer, J.G. and Webb, C.T., 2015. Using modelling to disentangle the relative contributions of zoonotic and anthroponotic transmission: The case of Lassa fever. *PLOS Neglected Tropical Diseases*, *9*(1), p.e3398.

Lowe, R., Coelho, C.A., Barcellos, C., Carvalho, M.S., Catao, R.D.C., Coelho, G.E., Ramalho, W.M., Bailey, T.C., Stephenson, D.B. and Rodo, X., 2016. Evaluating probabilistic dengue risk forecasts from a prototype early warning system for Brazil. *eLife*, *5*, p.e11285.

Lukashevich, I.S., Clegg, J.C.S. and Sidibe, K., 1993. Lassa virus activity in Guinea: Distribution of human antiviral antibody defined using enzyme-linked immunosorbent assay with recombinant antigen. *Journal of Medical Virology*, *40*(3), pp.210–217.

Massawe, A.W., Rwamugira, W., Leirs, H., Makundi, R.H. and Mulungu, L.S., 2007. Do farming practices influence population dynamics of rodents? A case study of the multimammate field rats, Mastomys natalensis, in Tanzania. *African Journal of Ecology*, *45*(3), pp.293–301.

Mateer, E.J., Huang, C., Shehu, N.Y. and Paessler, S., 2018. Lassa fever–induced sensorineural hearing loss: A neglected public health and social burden. *PLOS Neglected Tropical Diseases*, *12*(2), p.e0006187.

Mayrhuber, E.A.S., Niederkrotenthaler, T. and Kutalek, R., 2017. "We are survivors and not a virus": Content analysis of media reporting on Ebola survivors in Liberia. *PLOS Neglected Tropical Diseases*, *11*(8), p.e0005845.

McCarthy, M., 2002. USA moves quickly to push biodefence research. *The Lancet*, *360*(9335), p.732.

McCormick, J.B., 1987. Epidemiology and control of Lassa fever. In *Arenaviruses* (pp. 69–78). Berlin, Heidelberg: Springer.

McCormick, J.B., King, I.J., Webb, P.A., Johnson, K.M., O'Sullivan, R., Smith, E.S., Trippel, S. and Tong, T.C., 1987. A case-control study of the clinical diagnosis and course of Lassa fever. *Journal of Infectious Diseases*, *155*(3), pp.445–455.

Nigeria Center for Disease Control (NCDC), 2012. Weekly epidemiological report. *Wer Nigeria, 2*(18). http://www.fmh.gov.ng/images/stories/documents/WeeklyEpidemiologyReport_FMOH_11th_May_2012.pdf.

Nigeria Center for Disease Control (NCDC), 2016. First annual report of the Nigeria centre for disease control. http://www.ncdc.gov.ng/themes/common/docs/protocols/78_1515412191.pdf.

Nigeria Center for Disease Control (NCDC), 2018. National guidelines for Lassa fever case management, 30 November 2018.

Nigeria Center for Disease Control (NCDC), 2020. Lassa fever situation report, 12 April 2020.

Nigeria Center for Disease Control (NCDC), 2022. Lassa fever situation report. Week 8: 21–27 February 2022.

Ogbu, O., Ajuluchukwu, E. and Uneke, C.J., 2007. Lassa fever in West African sub-region: An overview. *Journal of Vector Borne Diseases*, *44*(1), pp.1–11.

Olayemi, A., Obadare, A., Oyeyiola, A., Fasogbon, S., Igbokwe, J., Igbahenah, F., Ortsega, D., Günther, S., Verheyen, E. and Fichet-Calvet, E., 2018. Small mammal diversity and dynamics within Nigeria, with emphasis on reservoirs of the Lassa virus. *Systematics and Biodiversity*, *16*(2), pp.118–127.

Olayemi, A., Obadare, A., Oyeyiola, A., Igbokwe, J., Fasogbon, A., Igbahenah, F., Ortsega, D., Asogun, D., Umeh, P., Vakkai, I. and Abejegah, C., 2016. Arenavirus diversity and phylogeography of Mastomys natalensis rodents, Nigeria. *Emerging Infectious Diseases*, *22*(4), pp. 694–697.

Omilabu, S.A., Badaru, S.O., Okokhere, P., Asogun, D., Drosten, C., Emmerich, P., Becker-Ziaja, B., Schmitz, H. and Günther, S., 2005. Lassa fever, Nigeria, 2003 and 2004. *Emerging Infectious Diseases*, *11*(10), pp.1642–1644.

Oppliger, J., Torriani, G., Herrador, A. and Kunz, S., 2016. Lassa virus cell entry via dystroglycan involves an unusual pathway of macropinocytosis. *Journal of Virology*, *90*(14), pp.6412–6429.

Price, M.E., Fisher-Hoch, S.P., Craven, R.B. and McCormick, J.B., 1988. A prospective study of maternal and fetal outcome in acute Lassa fever infection during pregnancy. *British Medical Journal*, *297*(6648), pp.584–587.

Røttingen, J.A., Gouglas, D., Feinberg, M., Plotkin, S., Raghavan, K.V., Witty, A., Draghia-Akli, R., Stoffels, P. and Piot, P., 2017. New vaccines against epidemic infectious diseases. *New England Journal of Medicine*, *376*(7), pp.610–613.

Shaffer, J.G., Grant, D.S., Schieffelin, J.S., Boisen, M.L., Goba, A., Hartnett, J.N., Levy, D.C., Yenni, R.E., Moses, L.M., Fullah, M. and Momoh, M., 2014. Lassa fever in post-conflict Sierra Leone. *PLOS Neglected Tropical Diseases*, *8*(3), p.e2748.

Siddle, K.J., Eromon, P., Barnes, K.G., Mehta, S., Oguzie, J.U., Odia, I., Schaffner, S.F., Winnicki, S.M., Shah, R.R., Qu, J. and Wohl, S., 2018. Genomic analysis of Lassa virus during an increase in cases in Nigeria in 2018. *New England Journal of Medicine*, *379*(18), pp.1745–1753.

Sogoba, N., Rosenke, K., Adjemian, J., Diawara, S.I., Maiga, O., Keita, M., Konaté, D., Keita, A.S., Sissoko, I., Boisen, M. and Nelson, D., 2016. Lassa virus seroprevalence in sibirilia commune, Bougouni District, Southern Mali. *Emerging Infectious Diseases*, *22*(4), pp.657–663.

Ter Meulen, J., Lenz, O., Koivogui, L., Magassouba, N.F., Kaushik, S.K., Lewis, R. and Aldis, W., 2001. Lassa fever in Sierra Leone: Un peacekeepers are at risk. *Tropical Medicine and International Health*, *6*(1), pp.83–84.

Ter Meulen, J., Lukashevich, I., Sidibe, K., Inapogui, A., Marx, M., Dorlemann, A., Yansane, M.L., Koulemou, K., Chang-Claude, J. and Schmitz, H., 1996. Hunting of peridomestic rodents and consumption of their meat as possible risk factors for rodent-to-human transmission of Lassa virus in the Republic of Guinea. *The American Journal of Tropical Medicine and Hygiene*, *55*(6), pp.661–666.

Tomori, O., Fabiyi, A., Sorungbe, A., Smith, A. and McCormick, J.B., 1988. Viral hemorrhagic fever antibodies in Nigerian populations. *The American Journal of Tropical Medicine and Hygiene*, *38*(2), pp.407–410.

UK Health Security Agency, 2014. Lassa fever: Origins, reservoirs, transmission and guidelines. http://www.giv.uk/guidiance/lassa-fever-origins-reservoirs-transmission-and-guidelines. Accessed on 5th March 2022.

Viral Haemorrhagic Fevers Consortium (VHFC), 2013. Viral haemorrhagic fevers consortium: Lassa fever. http://www.vhfc.org/lassa_fever.

Wilson, M.E., 1995. Infectious diseases: An ecological perspective. *BMJ*, *311*(7021), pp.1681–1684.

World Health Organization (WHO), 2019. *Lassa Fever.* Geneva, Switzerland: World Health Organization.

World Health Organization (WHO), 2022. Lassa fever-Nigeria. https://www.who.it/emergencies/disease-outbreak-news/item/lassa-fever---nigeria#:text=in%20Nigeria%2C%20frim%203%20to,the%20country%20(Figure%201).

Yun, N.E. and Walker, D.H., 2012. Pathogenesis of Lassa fever. *Viruses*, *4*(10), pp.2031–2048.

Zhao, S., Musa, S.S., Fu, H., He, D. and Qin, J., 2020. Large-scale Lassa fever outbreaks in Nigeria: Quantifying the association between disease reproduction number and local rainfall. *Epidemiology and Infection*, *148*, pp.1–12.

10 Contribution of Anthropogenic Factors to the Global Advancement of Zika Virus

Manika Vij, Sai Aditya Reddy Lingampally, and Saurabh Pandey

CONTENTS

10.1 Introduction 152
10.2 Historical Overview 153
10.3 Spatial and Temporal Progression of Zika Virus 153
10.4 Possible Routes of Viral Transmission 154
10.5 Clinical Implications of the Disease 155
10.6 Diagnostics and ZIKV Infection 155
10.7 Factors Leading to the Emergence of Zika 156
10.7.1 Temperature 156
10.7.1.1 Optimal Temperatures for ZIKV Infection Spread 157
10.7.2 Rainfall 158
10.7.3 Socio-Economic Status 158
10.7.4 Evolution 159
10.7.5 Possibility of Spillback from Humans to Animals (Urban to Zoonotic Cycle) in Areas Outside Africa 160
10.7.6 Insufficient Knowledge of Host Reservoirs for ZIKV 160
10.7.7 Poor Characterisation of the Spectrum of Species Involved in the Transmission Cycle 161
10.7.8 Role of Vector Capacity in an Outbreak 161
10.7.9 Contribution of Vertical/Venereal Transmission 161
10.8 Proposed Control Methods for ZIKV-Mediated Disease 162
10.8.1 Use of Wolbachia-Incorporated Mosquitoes as an Effective Strategy 162
10.8.2 Model-Based Prediction of the Sylvatic Spread 163
10.8.3 Vaccines 163

DOI: 10.1201/9781003288732-10

10.8.4 Milk ... 164
10.8.5 Mathematical Models to Predict the Dynamics of ZIKV Spread and How It Can Affect the Future of an Epidemic ... 164
10.9 Conclusion ... 164
References ... 165

10.1 INTRODUCTION

Viruses are sub-microscopic entities that possess the unique ability to survive inside living cells. They can either utilise the host's replication machinery to multiply and cause infection or might remain dormant for years, depending upon the environmental cues. Depending upon their genetic material, these organisms can be classified as DNA/RNA-based viruses having a single- or double-stranded genome. This genetic material of a virus is usually encapsulated within a protective protein coat termed a capsid. However, in some cases, it may have small, well-organised units on its surface, which may or may not be accompanied by the surrounding envelope (Mateu, 2013). Viral infections are usually difficult to treat and might lead to long-term health impairment. Commonly available antibiotics do not help alleviate these infections; therefore, developing effective antiviral medicines or vaccines is a prerequisite. Apart from the general health status of an individual, many other environmental or abiotic factors, such as temperature, rainfall, vector–host inhabitation, and urbanisation, can contribute to the dissemination of viral infections. In this chapter, we attempt to understand how these anthropogenic factors affect life-threatening viral outbreaks and what control measures can be implemented to avoid epidemics/pandemics and achieve partial or complete protection from such hazardous outcomes.

Flaviviruses are a class of positive, single-stranded, enveloped RNA viruses that can survive in arthropods and may infect humans. Yellow fever, West Nile virus, Japanese encephalitis, tick-borne encephalitis virus, Powassan virus, and dengue virus all belong to this family of arboviruses. These organisms are well known to cause severe diseases in humans, such as yellow fever, dengue, encephalitis, and hepatitis C, to name a few (Gutiérrez-Bugallo et al., 2019; Yadav et al., 2016). Another important member of this class of viruses and the concern of our chapter is the Zika virus. In February 2016, post epidemic, the WHO declared Zika virus (ZIKV) dissemination as a public health emergency of international concern. Due to its association with the manifestation of various neurological and congenital complications, the virus was considered detrimental to humans. Moreover, it could lead to many life-threatening congenital disabilities and long-term disabilities (Calvet et al., 2016), which are difficult to treat. In this chapter, we specifically discuss the spatial and temporal emergence and evolution of the Zika virus, list various anthropogenic factors that might have assisted in its global dissemination, and propose effective measures or strategies to control such outbreaks and prevent the occurrence of a Zika pandemic as a future outcome.

10.2 HISTORICAL OVERVIEW

Briefly, in 1947, ZIKV was first discovered in a sentinel rhesus macaque that was captured from the Zika forest of Uganda for routine surveillance of yellow fever. One year later, this virus was also isolated from the *Aedes* (*Stegomyia*) *africanus* mosquito obtained from the same forest area, indicating it to be an arbovirus. Furthermore, the first human case of ZIKV was reported in 1952, when serological testing recorded the presence of antibodies in individuals inhabiting these areas (Gutiérrez-Bugallo et al., 2019; Musso et al., 2019). So, how this virus residing in such a remote location disseminated over many continents, thereby leading to multiple epidemics, needs thorough investigation. It will be interesting to know if arthropods are the major transporters of this virus or if other factors contribute to its widespread presence. In the upcoming section, we mention how ZIKV spread occurred in different parts of the world over time.

10.3 SPATIAL AND TEMPORAL PROGRESSION OF ZIKA VIRUS

Until 2007, two genetically distinct strains of ZIKV belonging to the African and Asian lineages initiated sporadic infections with mild clinical manifestations in people in Africa and Southeast Asia. Meanwhile, it was also directly detected in other regions like Senegal, Ivory Coast, Burkina Faso, Nigeria, Central African Republic, Thailand, Malaysia, Indonesia, and the Philippines. But, the first major outbreak of ZIKV infection in Gabon and Yap (2007) immediately diverted attention towards controlling its spread (Figure 10.1). It was hypothesised that a viraemic individual from the Philippines introduced this spread. This large-scale outbreak was followed by another major spread of ZIKV infection (Asian lineage) in French Polynesia (2013), which affected >100,000 individuals and provided the first evidence of Guillain–Barré syndrome. Due to extensive air travel, the virus spread eastwards and westwards, ultimately entering local regions within America. This gave rise to an enormous ZIKV epidemic in 2015 in Brazil. The presence of El Niño further helped in the advancement of the epidemic's after-effects. In addition to extensive air travel, other introduction events hypothesised to be linked to this epidemic were the Soccer World Cup 2014, the World Spring Canoe Championship 2014, and the Confederations Cup (15–30 June) 2013. It was mentioned that due to these events, Brazil witnessed a lot of movement and travel from outsiders who might be coming from ZIKV risk zones, leading to the spread of virus infection. Around the same time, in February 2014, indigenous ZIKV was reported on Easter Island (Chile) in the South Pacific (America). Lineage identification of this indigenous strain revealed it to be a completely new American strain, spreading further eastwards to affect Cape Verde and other regions. In 2016, Caribbean islands also reported independent cases of ZIKV infection. By 2017, 48 countries reported the presence of ZIKV (Depoux et al., 2018; Gutiérrez-Bugallo et al., 2019; Yadav et al., 2016). Later, millions of cases with the manifestation of an expanded form of these syndromes were reported from 86 countries. Moreover, extensive patient studies revealed, for the first time, an association of

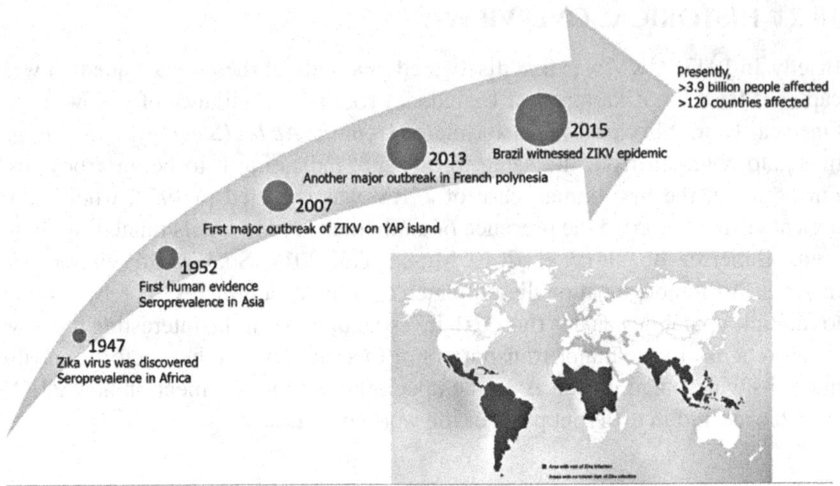

FIGURE 10.1 Historical spread of the Zika virus.

congenital microencephaly with maternal ZIKV infections. Presently, more than 3.9 billion people in 120 countries are affected by the ZIKV infection, making it a medical emergency. But, how this endemic transformed into an epidemic and what factors determined this switch need to be considered. This will not only help us to understand the spreading trend of this virus but also help in predicting its predilection towards pandemics.

10.4 POSSIBLE ROUTES OF VIRAL TRANSMISSION

Before we delve into details of how this ubiquitous presence of the virus occurred, it is essential to know its possible transmission routes from one region to another. Most viruses, in general, exhibit an arboreal mode of transmission whereby a final mosquito bite in humans leads to the horizontal transfer. The two species of mosquito that act as vectors for ZIKV are *Aedes aegypti* and *Aedes albopictus*. They are known to aid in active infection and the spread of ZIKV to humans. However, sometimes other members of this family, such as *Ae. africanus*, *Ae. luteocephalus*, *Ae. vitattus*, *Ae. furcifer*, *Ae. hensilii*, and *Ae. apicoargenteus*, might also lead to viral spread.

Furthermore, other species of mosquitoes, for example, the Culex family, are also known to cause active transmission of ZIKV (Chouin-Carneiro et al., 2016; Gutiérrez-Bugallo et al., 2019). Various research studies show that usually, it is the abundance of a particular vector in a specific geographical location that determines its potential to act as a major transmitter of ZIKV infection. What has been more intriguing is the presence of viral particles in novel arthropods usually found in city dwellings. This highlights the impressive adaptation potential of both viruses and harbouring insects, which may lead to the spread of more epidemics or pandemics in the future. In addition to the arboreal spread, other routes of ZIKV transmission also exist. It can be transmitted sexually, through laboratory-acquired infections, through transfusion of blood products, or by in utero/perinatal transmission from mother to child (Depoux et al., 2018; Musso et al., 2019). Breastfeeding is also assumed to play a role in transmitting the Zika virus from mother to child. But due to the presence of essential nutritional components in mother's milk, the WHO issued guidelines to ensure that these mothers still feed their babies. Similarly, multiple experimental and clinical studies have shown the presence of ZIKV RNA in colostrum 14 days post infection and even up to 32 days post infection (dpi). However, limited evidence of actual infections in infants that are specifically due to feeding and not vector-borne makes it difficult to formulate any general conclusion in this direction (Mann et al., 2019). Another rapid mode of transmission of ZIKV disease is extensive air travel. Individuals who frequently fly to outbreak-affected zones most of the time bring the virus back to their place of origin. When this virus finds a conducive environment to grow, it starts inhabiting other vector–host cells and initiates the viral spread along with the manifestation of disease in later stages.

10.5 CLINICAL IMPLICATIONS OF THE DISEASE

Post transmission into humans, viral particles can lead to multiple clinical complications that range from mild to severe. Primarily, ZIKV infection is often mild and asymptomatic in nature. Clinically, it manifests in the form of mild fever (37–38 °C), stiffness of small joints (hands and feet), headache, muscular weakness, retro-orbital pain, conjunctivitis, and cutaneous maculopapular rash on the trunk and extremities. Sometimes, symptoms of active ZIKV infection resemble influenza, which might lead to incorrect diagnosis. Blood examination of these individuals also reveals a decrease in leukocytes and platelets and an increase in the total number of blood lymphocytes. A more severe or grave form of the disease involves neurological complications collectively termed Guillain–Barré syndrome. In infants, ZIKV infection often leads to microcephaly and long-term congenital disabilities. Pregnant women with ZIKV infection undergo miscarriages or may give birth to still-born babies (Calvet et al., 2016; Gutiérrez-Bugallo et al., 2019; Pan American Health Organization, 2016). The absence of defined and specifically associated clinical symptoms makes it difficult to diagnose a Zika infection, one of the major lacunae in timely control of this infection.

10.6 DIAGNOSTICS AND ZIKV INFECTION

Early and precise diagnosis of ZIKV infection is challenging and important to curb its infection rate and after-infection effects in humans. Overlapping clinical features with other flu-like viruses make it difficult to identify the infection phenotypically, i.e., through patient symptoms only. Therefore, in addition to early reporting of ZIKV infection by the patient and their thorough check-up by the doctor, proper and time-efficient testing at a biochemical and molecular level is also required to confirm the presence of viral particles. Both government health agencies and non-governmental organisations play a major role in helping to spread awareness and the need for early reporting of such infections in order to control them effectively without delay.

Present methods of tracing ZIKV infections in humans involve reverse transcriptase- polymerase chain reaction (RT-PCR)-based detection of its amplified genetic material in the blood and other body fluids such as saliva, urine, and semen. In addition, amniotic fluid or umbilical cord are used for testing purposes for pregnant females. Another alternative detection method involves the investigation of IgM antibodies in the serum of patients' blood using enzyme-linked immunosorbent assay (ELISA) (Calvet et al., 2016). However, despite continuous testing, low viral load, and cross-reactivity with other flaviviruses, it becomes challenging to interpret these diagnostic results and avoid misdiagnosis. Hence, there is still a need for a better, rapid, and cheaper method that is more sensitive and specific for detecting ZIKV.

An independent study showed that patient urine has much higher titres of virus present from 1 week onwards post onset of infection, and the virus can be detected for longer periods as compared with serum samples. Moreover, it is a non-invasive and easy-to-use method, thereby encouraging it as a testing material for rapid testing in frequent travellers (Gourinat et al., 2015). Moreover, with advancements in microfluidics-based devices, the development of many low-cost, specific, sensitive, and efficient kits is underway, and these will be used for large-scale testing and diagnosis in the future (Herrada et al., 2018).

10.7 FACTORS LEADING TO THE EMERGENCE OF ZIKA

Apart from virus–host interaction and proper diagnostic procedures, other well-known environmental and socio-economic factors can also influence the spread of endemic and epidemic ZIKV globally (Figure 10.2). However, the lack of key information regarding potential novel viral hosts and vectors and possible transmission conditions has mainly contributed to the failure to predict or control its outbreaks efficiently. Here, we list some of the significant factors that influence the spread of infection as well as the survival of the virus to maintain its long-term reservoirs.

10.7.1 Temperature

Temperature is an important factor that influences the spread of various vector-borne diseases. Mosquitoes are ectothermic organisms that exhibit a unimodal response to temperature in the life cycle, physiology, and vectorial capacity context. Therefore, they exhibit ideal growth, survival, and infection conditions at a single optimum temperature value. But, how this effect of temperature variation on the mosquito cycle will influence the ZIKV infection rate remains elusive. Therefore, a sincere effort to study this parameter experimentally in laboratory or field trials will not only help us to find an explanation for the epidemics that occurred in the past but also predict further spreading trends and the possibility of ZIKV becoming a pandemic in a temperature-dependent manner.

In the past few years, various empirical and mathematical models have been designed to predict the effect of environmental factors on ZIKV infection/transmission. However, limited understanding of a vector–pathogen relationship with environmental factors, pre-assumption of ZIKV being the same as dengue virus, and the use of a poor quality and quantity of data vastly impede the accuracy of the outcomes of these models.

Murdock et al. studied the effect of temperature variation on ZIKV transmission using a field-derived *Aedes aegypti*. They observed the unimodal impact of temperature on vector competence, external incubation period, and survival, as mentioned before. Using these results, they improvised an existing thermal model. They predicted optimal temperature values (as mentioned in the following subsection) that will enhance ZIKV transmission, increase dissemination of viral particles within the mosquito, support rapid expectoration of the virus into the environment, and improve mosquito survival for sustainable infections.

10.7.1.1 Optimal Temperatures for ZIKV Infection Spread

a) Maximal transmission by *Aedes aegypti*: 29 °C (22.7 to 34.7 °C)
b) Maximal vector competence: 30.6 °C (22.9 to 38.4 °C)

This reveals that temperatures lower than 30.6 °C may lead to poor dissemination of viral particles from the mosquito's mid-gut to other organs. Temperatures higher than 30.6 °C might support infection increase but in later stages will definitely lead to mortality of mosquitoes, thereby preventing the spread of infection and lowering vector competence.

c) Extrinsic incubation period: 36.4 °C (19.7 to 42.5 °C)

This is the time the virus takes to travel from the mid-gut to the salivary gland of mosquitoes, following which it can be expectorated into the environment. Warmer temperatures usually decrease the extrinsic incubation period, leading to faster dissemination of infection. In experimental data, it was evident that there was no infection even after 21 dpi at 16 °C, compared with 38 °C, where the infection was observed at 3 dpi.

d) Vector survival: 24° C

This is the ideal temperature for mosquito survival. However, as per research studies, temperatures between 36 and 38 °C are high enough to cause increased mosquito mortality, thereby constraining transmission potential.

Thus, any shift in temperatures due to extensive global warming, urbanisation, or seasonality can help expand ZIKV in northern regions and into longer seasons. A similar trend has also been observed for malaria in Ethiopian and Columbian highlands, where its spread is increasing due to rising temperatures. Also, places with optimal temperatures may not be suitable locations for epidemics over time. Hence, accurate estimation of optimal temperature is paramount in predicting where climate warming will expand, contract, or shift the transmission potential.

Temperature prediction also highlights the difference in thermal minimum for ZIKV transmission, which is 5 °C warmer than for dengue virus, thereby clearly demarcating the preferred locations for their respective transmission (Tesla et al., 2018).

In another independent study, two mosquito species obtained from temperate regions were investigated, and the minimum transmission threshold from these vectors was predicted as 17 to 19 °C, which is 10 degrees lower than for the tropics, as mentioned before. The R0-thermal model in this study predicts that ZIKV transmission will increase over southern and eastern Europe, the northern USA, and temperate regions of Asia in future climate conditions (Blagrove et al., 2020). Although these models can be really useful to predict the disease dynamics, they still suffer from certain limitations, such as non-inclusion of the effect of the genetic background of the vector and infecting pathogen, or other abiotic factors like rainfall, humidity, biotic factors, and socio-economic factors, which can also influence the outcomes.

10.7.2 Rainfall

The larval stages of *Aedes aegypti*, a well-known arthropod vector for ZIKV, require shallow pools of water to grow. Therefore, a few weeks of abundant rainfall could be ideal for these mosquitoes to breed and increase their numbers to spread epidemic infections. As per reports, the time lag after rain is crucial in deciding mosquito breeding and abundance. However, heavy rainfall can completely wipe out breeding hotspots, thereby preventing mosquito-borne infections from spreading immediately after the rainfall. Nevertheless, after 2–3 weeks, the larvae start developing in small water pools accumulated in walls, tyre holes, or any other cracks and crevices and grow abundantly in these unnoticed areas, thereby increasing the dissemination of sudden infections. A similar effect was observed in October 2015 when there were heavy rains from September 2015 to early October 2015, followed by the ZIKV epidemic from the end of October 2015 up to December 2015 (Rees et al., 2018) in Brazil.

10.7.3 Socio-Economic Status

Vector occurrence is often determined by various climatic and environmental factors influencing its abundance and activity. Although this is a major determinant for the spread of ZIKV infection, another significant factor is the host dwelling conditions and social status. Those mostly affected are humans living in poor areas with low-quality housing facilities, for example, no window screen protection, poor sanitation and hygiene, non-availability of proper healthcare facilities, and insufficient nutrition, leading to compromised immunity and ability to fight infections. All these factors increase the risk of such individuals being exposed to infected vectors, missing out on early diagnosis and appropriate treatment options, and remaining carriers. In addition, the high mobility of these groups into pathogen-free areas can influence infection outcomes. Densely populated areas usually have better infection detection rates due to proper healthcare facilities and careful surveillance systems. Hence, population dynamics can help predict the rate of infection occurrence in pathogen-free areas. A recent study used logistic regression and Virus-based (accelerated failure time) models to predict vector abundance and population dynamics as indicators of ZIKV infection emergence. Another social factor includes a lack of education and awareness regarding reporting and treating health disorders in impoverished areas. This primarily affects the modelling outcomes, as cases not reported often lead to a negative correlation between poverty and infection in such areas, thereby leading to misrepresentation of correct information (Rees et al., 2018).

Furthermore, improved aviation and global connectivity have also contributed to the spread of ZIKV infection. Individuals travelling to risk zones have managed to transmit these infected vectors in new habitats, where they increase resistance to environmental conditions and improvise themselves genetically to survive and expedite the spread of large-scale infections. Thus, urban practices have also been instrumental in enhancing the spread of ZIKV worldwide.

In the past few years, increased urbanisation and rapid loss of animals' natural habitat have forced them to dwell close to human-inhabited areas, thereby increasing the possibility of transmission in urban settings and enhancing human–mosquito contact, which can undoubtedly aid in the spread of infections. This can also explain the explosive nature of recent outbreaks where the vector might have undergone genetic alterations in urban areas, affecting its pathogenicity or aiding its efficient and widespread transmission to domesticated animals and humans, creating large-scale future reservoirs and finally causing epidemics (Fuller et al., 2017), as emphasised in the following two sections.

10.7.4 Evolution

Asia and Africa witnessed the spread of ZIKV by two completely genetically different strains. The Asian ZIKV strain extended outwards to the Pacific Ocean and was responsible for the outbreak in 2007 on the Yap island, followed by Guam and Micronesia. Around 2013–2014, the virus was also introduced into French Polynesia and other islands. Due to extensive air travel, the virus eventually entered the mainland in May 2015, leading to a massive outbreak in Brazil, further supported by El Niño. Later, it entered Central and Southern America and the Caribbean (Gutiérrez-Bugallo et al., 2019). This constant movement of the virus from one region to another possibly helped in its adaptation towards being transmitted by various locally existing urban vectors and improved infectivity, thereby leading to continuous outbreaks from then on.

10.7.5 Possibility of Spillback from Humans to Animals (Urban to Zoonotic Cycle) in Areas Outside Africa

Further, what might explain the sudden outbreak of ZIKV in many urban and rural settings of America is the possible spillback of ZIKV from humans and the establishment of an enzootic cycle. This depends on host–vector population size, interaction competence, host birth rate, and vector infectivity rate. However, to rule out spillback from the natural enzootic cycle, it is important to study the host competence of New World primates, the vector competence of New World mosquitoes, the geographical range of each of these, and epizootics in non-human primates, as well as to distinguish differences between animal and human strains. These explorations could have important implications for the ultimate control of future epidemics, as these cycles are not amenable to human intervention and control (Althouse et al., 2016). If the spillback theory is true, then this close inhabitation of animals and humans could lead to a never-ending vicious cycle of ZIKV circulation and large-scale infections, which might be too difficult to control.

10.7.6 Insufficient Knowledge of Host Reservoirs for ZIKV

In addition to mosquitoes, vertebrate animals constitute a significant resource for maintaining ZIKV. As observed in Africa, this is highly evident from sylvatic transmission between non-human primate animals and arboreal mosquitoes. This serologically apparent enzootic amplification occurs in a continuous cycle where the virus is detected every 4 years, unlike other viruses, which take 7–8 years. ZIKV often shows a predilection towards short-lived vertebrate hosts having a fast turnover. Such animal studies outside Africa are still lacking. Only Brazil, Thailand, Indonesia, and Pakistan have looked into this factor. Therefore, it is essential to develop appropriate diagnostic techniques to identify which zoonotic species can maintain sufficient virus titres to cause viraemia and infect mosquitoes, ensuring natural circulation and promoting never-ending outbreaks. Mammals, especially primates, are the most represented taxonomic group, although birds, reptiles, and amphibians have also been identified, indicating the potential diversity of ZIKV hosts and the lack of a clear association between ZIKV and a particular animal taxon. The incrimination of such animals in ZIKV transmission chains (either sylvatic or urban) will depend on their viraemia levels and duration, their spatial coincidence with competent ZIKV vectors, and the feeding preferences of the latter. So far, viraemia levels sufficient for transmission have been detected in five monkey species (*Macaca mulatta*, *Callithrix jacchus*, *Macaca fascicularis*, *Saimiri boliviensis boliviensis*, and *Saimiri sciureus sciureus*), which were infected experimentally. However, the field data regarding appropriate host reservoirs are still unknown (Gutiérrez-Bugallo et al., 2019).

10.7.7 Poor Characterisation of the Spectrum of Species Involved in the Transmission Cycle

Mosquitoes infected by ZIKV have been mainly classified into five major genera: Aedes, Culex, Anopheles, Eretmapodites, and Mansonia. Out of these, Aedes is the major taxon responsible for ZIKV transmission. Usually, ZIKV can be transmitted in either sylvatic or urban settings, thereby passing on infection to wild or domesticated animals. The first category majorly involves *Ae. africanus*, *Ae. furcifer*, *Ae. lutocephalus*, *Ae. vittatus*, *Ae. dalzielli*, and *Ae. taylori*. However, urban transmission mainly occurs in *Ae. aegypti*. This is evident from the anthropophilic and anthropophagic nature of this mosquito, which mainly inhabits the tropics and is present in abundance.

In a laboratory study, *Ae. vittatus* and *Ae. luteocephalus* were found to be competent ZIKV vectors, also evident from their high frequency and distribution in fields in Africa, thereby explaining the sylvatic spread in the region. However, a similar study with urban strains *Ae* (*Stegomyia*) *hensilli* or *polynesiensis*, prevalent in households of Yap island and French Polynesia outbreaks, revealed that these strains could not transmit the virus despite being infected. Moreover, they were also absent in the field trial studies in these regions, highlighting the need for further investigation in this direction.

Therefore, it is important to understand that any transmission, urban or sylvatic, requires proper interaction between host and vector. Furthermore, the vector may also be a carrier of residual infection and may not always indicate an active viral infection. Often, a vector is infected and disseminated but still shows a low infection rate. Hence, these data are imperative to list possible ZIKV vectors that can cause active infection by these two transmission routes, also known as vector competence (Gutiérrez-Bugallo et al., 2019).

10.7.8 Role of Vector Capacity in an Outbreak

Vectorial capacity also plays a crucial role in causing an outbreak. It is defined as the abundance of a vector and its ecological traits, which increase the chances of spreading infection in an urban setting. For example, the Culex mosquito *Cx. quinquefasciatus* is present in large numbers in urban areas, naturally increasing its interaction with the host. As a result, it can bite humans more frequently and lead to occasional ZIKV infections. However, since this species is often associated with avian blood meal, it has been ruled out as a major causative agent of ZIKV infections. But, other mosquitoes in abundance in urban areas or having migrated from forests to cities due to excessive deforestation can certainly become new spreaders of ZIKV infection.

10.7.9 Contribution of Vertical/Venereal Transmission

During dormant conditions like harsh weather, severe drought, and herd immunity during the inter-epidemic phase, the viruses maintain themselves by vertical transmission from mothers to offspring (evidence of virus obtained from eggs). Additionally, they exhibit venereal transmission from male to female and vice versa, leading to continuous presence and inter-vector virus transmission. However, whether this maintenance contributes to vector–host transmission or active infections is a significant lacuna that needs to be filled with further investigations.

Although such studies are still underway, many other methods have been proposed and are being used in field trials to control the spread of ZIKV infection (Figure 10.2). However, further validations and field trials are needed to discover whether these methods can contribute significantly in this direction.

10.8 PROPOSED CONTROL METHODS FOR ZIKV-MEDIATED DISEASE

10.8.1 Use of Wolbachia-Incorporated Mosquitoes as an Effective Strategy

ZIKV is not only a mosquito-borne disease but also a global public health emergency. Due to its associated neurological and congenital damage, it is imperative to control the spread of this virus and avoid future outbreaks. One way of preventing ZIKV spread is to control its vector. Traditional methods used to control mosquitoes include using chemicals like insecticides that can kill both larvae and

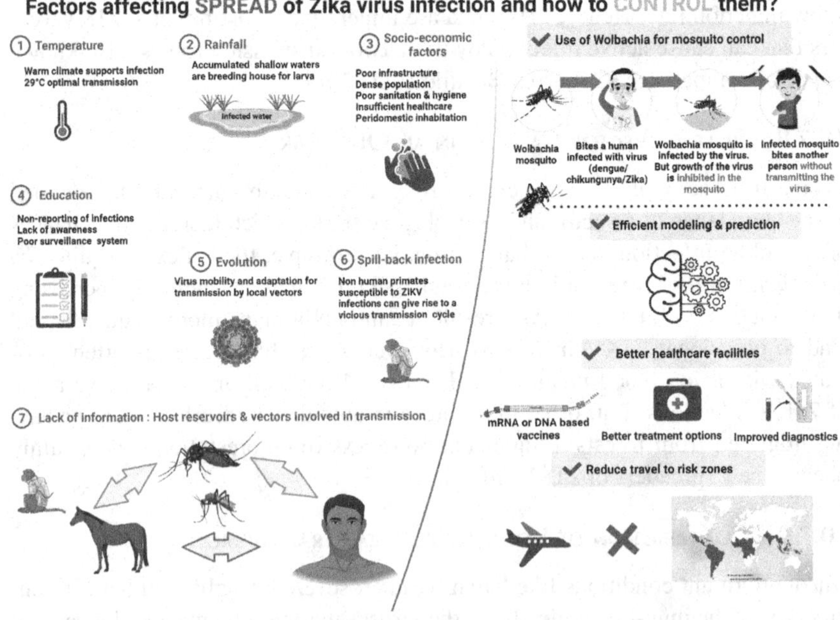

FIGURE 10.2 Factors causing ZIKV infection and their effective control measures.

adult forms, removal of source containers where mosquitoes can breed actively, such as tyres or water-filled containers, and changes in environmental factors, such as the use of a subsoil drainage system. However, these traditional mosquito control methods are being supplanted by a novel biological method using the endosymbiotic *Wolbachia pipientis*. Other bacteria such as *Bacillus thuringiensis israelensis* (Bti) and *Bacillus sphaericus* (Bs) or organisms like fish have been used for similar purposes but with limited potential. *Wolbachia* has already been shown to effectively block or reduce infection with various pathogens such as yellow fever virus, dengue virus, chikungunya, and plasmodium in mosquitoes of different species, indicating its immense potential to control mosquito-borne diseases in humans. In Brazil, the wMel strain of *Wolbachia* has successfully blocked the spread of ZIKV infection by preventing the transmission of infectious viral particles in mosquito saliva. It has been hypothesised that the presence of this bacterium in the vector leads to decreased replication of virus, reduction in cell invasion, and increased extrinsic incubation period, thereby delaying the transmission rate, preventing viral exit from the mid-gut, and resulting in poor expectorant ability in mosquitoes infected with the bacterium. Moreover, it spreads actively within the mosquitoes due to cytoplasmic incompatibility without affecting host competitiveness and simultaneously offering a high degree of viral inhibition. Despite these advantages, one major limitation of *Wolbachia* is that it takes a long time to establish within the mosquito. Hence, it can be used as a preventive measure for long-term effects and not as a method to control actively ongoing ZIKV infection. Other unanswered questions include whether this bacterium will behave similarly in varying environmental conditions and whether it will be universally effective against all genotypes of ZIKV to serve as an effective control measure (Caragata et al., 2016).

10.8.2 Model-Based Prediction of the Sylvatic Spread

Residence of non-human primates close to humans emphasises the need to know their susceptibility to ZIKV infections. If these animals become infected, they can carry on with the enzootic cycle and transmit the virus to humans, giving rise to a never-ending vicious circle. If this sylvatic cycle is established, it will be challenging to eradicate this virus using conventional mosquito control methods or vaccinations. Hence, it is important to develop models using quality data to better predict the possibility of sylvatic spread in an area. Also, one should investigate the possible vectors that can serve as hosts for the virus and their differential ability to transmit disease across animals and humans. Presently, Aedes seems to be the global vector most likely to lead to sylvatic spread in urban areas due to its invasive nature and widespread presence in the tropics and temperate regions.

10.8.3 Vaccines

Despite a large number of incidences and available information on the pattern and prevalence of ZIKV infection, there is no specific treatment or vaccine available for this disease. However, efforts are being made to develop some DNA/mRNA-based vaccines along with attenuated viral strains, which could be used as vaccines against ZIKV infection. However, all these developments are in the preliminary phases of clinical trials and will take time to be ready for human use (Pattnaik et al., 2020). Hence, the WHO presently recommends that all travellers to ZIKV infection zones be cautious and vigilant about the disease to avoid its spread.

10.8.4 Milk

Since transmission of ZIKV from mothers to infants is sometimes evident, we must support using replacement feeds. A similar approach is also taken in the case of mothers infected with *Mycobacterium tuberculosis* or human immunodeficiency virus – type I.

10.8.5 Mathematical Models to Predict the Dynamics of ZIKV Spread and How It Can Affect the Future of an Epidemic

A recent study considered virus transmission with sexual contact and migration. According to these models, sexual transmission can only determine the magnitude and duration of a persistent infection; however, migration is the major deciding factor that regulates disease spread. After an outbreak, some residual infection always remains in an area. Now, when uni-directional migration happens to a new susceptible area, a low level of infection starts, leading to endemic low-intensity infection in both regions. However, bi-directional migration between these two areas leads to the synchronisation of endemic infections at the two places over time, thus eventually giving rise to an epidemic. Hence, it is important to control movement from outbreak-affected regions to other susceptible regions to control the spread of ZIKV (Baca-Carrasco and Velasco-Hernández, 2016). From 2007 to 2013, few cases were reported in travellers from Africa and Southeast Asia. Moreover, sexual transmission of the disease is more prominent in women; hence, using condoms or avoiding movement of pregnant females to ZIKV-affected zones can help alleviate the viral infection.

In addition to these control measures, the development of accurate predictive models, better recording of surveillance data, provision of better health facilities, and following hygienic practices are some of the general factors that can aid in successfully curbing ZIKV infections.

10.9 CONCLUSION

Zika virus has been known for many years, but it was declared a public health emergency by the WHO only after its first severe outbreak in Brazil. It largely affects pregnant females and fetuses, leading to neurological complications and auto-immune disorders. The development of an effective vaccine against this virus is still lacking. Therefore, secondary treatment in a complications-specific manner is the only remedy. Many molecular and serological tests have been devised to diagnose ZIKV infection; however, increased cross-reactivity with other members of flaviviruses and low sensitivity vastly impede their widespread use. This, in turn, leads to misdiagnosis as one of the major lacunae of the disease. In addition to poor treatment regimes and improper diagnosis, the absence of awareness and delay in timely reporting of the disease also contribute to its increased presence among the population.

Recently, many researchers have been trying to elucidate the role of abiotic factors in supporting the dissemination of ZIKV infection. They have shown how various parameters such as temperature, rainfall, population density, migration rate, and vector–host interactions can alter the rate of infection. Moreover, they highlight the seriousness of this virus entering the enzootic and sylvatic cycle, whereupon controlling it by conventional methods could be impossible.

Many models have been proposed and are continuously being improvised to predict the future movement of the disease and prevent unwanted sudden outbreaks. Various biological and lifestyle-based control measures proposed in the last section of this chapter can help alleviate this life-damaging viral disease. With the advancement of microfluidics, efforts are being made to develop better, cost-effective, scalable, and efficient diagnostic kits for early disease detection. In addition, the latest DNA/RNA-based vaccine technology is being tested to develop an effective means of controlling infection in humans soon.

REFERENCES

Althouse, B. M., Vasilakis, N., Sall, A. A., Diallo, M., Weaver, S. C., & Hanley, K. A. (2016). Potential for zika virus to establish a sylvatic transmission cycle in the Americas. *PLOS Neglected Tropical Diseases*, *10*(12), 1–11. https://doi.org/10.1371/journal.pntd.0005055.

Baca-Carrasco, D., & Velasco-Hernández, J. X. (2016). Sex, mosquitoes and epidemics: An evaluation of zika disease dynamics. *Bulletin of Mathematical Biology*, *78*(11), 2228–2242. https://doi.org/10.1007/s11538-016-0219-4.

Blagrove, M. S. C., Caminade, C., Diggle, P. J., Patterson, E. I., Sherlock, K., Chapman, G. E., Hesson, J., Metelmann, S., McCall, P. J., Lycett, G., Medlock, J., Hughes, G. L., Della Torre, A., & Baylis, M. (2020). Potential for Zika virus transmission by mosquitoes in temperate climates: Zika transmission in temperate climates. *Proceedings of the Royal Society. Series B,: Biological Sciences*, *287*(1930). https://doi.org/10.1098/rspb.2020.0119rspb20200119.

Calvet, G. A., Dos Santos, F. B., & Sequeira, P. C. (2016). Zika virus infection: Epidemiology, clinical manifestations and diagnosis. *Current Opinion in Infectious Diseases*, *29*(5), 459–466. https://doi.org/10.1097/QCO.0000000000000301.

Caragata, E. P., Dutra, H. L. C., & Moreira, L. A. (2016). Inhibition of Zika virus by Wolbachia in Aedes aegypti. *Microbial Cell*, *3*(7), 293–295. https://doi.org/10.15698/mic2016.07.513.

Chouin-Carneiro, T., Vega-Rua, A., Vazeille, M., Yebakima, A., Girod, R., Goindin, D., Dupont-Rouzeyrol, M., Lourenço-de-Oliveira, R., & Failloux, A. B. (2016). Differential Susceptibilities of Aedes aegypti and Aedes albopictus from the Americas to Zika Virus. *PLOS Neglected Tropical Diseases*, *10*(3), 1–11. https://doi.org/10.1371/journal.pntd.0004543.

Depoux, A., Philibert, A., Rabier, S., Philippe, H. J., Fontanet, A., & Flahault, A. (2018). A multi-faceted pandemic: A review of the state of knowledge on the Zika virus. *Public Health Reviews*, *39*(1), 1–12. https://doi.org/10.1186/s40985-018-0087-6.

Fuller, T. L., Calvet, G., Estevam, C. G., Angelo, J. R., Abiodun, G. J., Halai, U. A., De Santis, B., Sequeira, P. C., Araujo, E. M., Sampaio, S. A., De Mendonça, M. C. L., Fabri, A., Ribeiro, R. M., Harrigan, R., Smith, T. B., Gabaglia, C. R., Brasil, P., De Filippis, A. M. B., & Nielsen-Saines, K. (2017). Behavioral, climatic, and environmental risk factors for Zika and Chikungunya virus infections in Rio de Janeiro, Brazil, 2015–16. *Plos One*, *12*(11), 1–15. https://doi.org/10.1371/journal.pone.0188002.

Gourinat, A. C., O'Connor, O., Calvez, E., Goarant, C., & Dupont-Rouzeyrol, M. (2015). Detection of zika virus in urine. *Emerging Infectious Diseases*, *21*(1), 84–86. https://doi.org/10.3201/eid2101.140894.

Gutiérrez-Bugallo, G., Piedra, L. A., Rodriguez, M., Bisset, J. A., Lourenço-de-Oliveira, R., Weaver, S. C., Vasilakis, N., & Vega-Rúa, A. (2019). Vector-borne transmission and evolution of Zika virus. *Nature Ecology and Evolution*, *3*(4), 561–569. https://doi.org/10.1038/s41559-019-0836-z.

Herrada, C. A., Kabir, A., Altamirano, R., & Asghar, W. (2018). Advances in diagnostic methods for zika virus infection. *Journal of Medical Devices, Transactions of the ASME*, *12*(4). https://doi.org/10.1115/1.4041086.

Mann, T. Z., Haddad, L. B., Williams, T. R., Hills, S. L., Read, J. S., Dee, D. L., Dziuban, E. J., Jamieson, D. J., Honein, A., & Shapiro-Mendoza, C. K. (2019). Breast milk transmission of flaviviruses in the context of Zika virus: A systematic review. *HHS Public Access*, *32*(4), 358–368. https://doi.org/10.1111/ppe.12478.

Mateu, M. G. (2013). *Structure and Physics of Viruses* (Vol. 68). https://doi.org/10.1007/978-94-007-6552-8.

Musso, D., Ko, A. I., & Baud, D. (2019). Zika virus infection — After the pandemic. *New England Journal of Medicine*, *381*(15), 1444–1457. https://doi.org/10.1056/nejmra1808246.

Pan American Health Organization. (2016). *Epidemiological Update: Neurological Syndrome, Congenital Anomalies, and Zika Virus Infection*. World Health Organization, 1–8. January 17, 2016.

Pattnaik, A., Sahoo, B. R., & Pattnaik, A. K. (2020). *Current Status of Zika Virus Vaccines: Successes and Challenges*, 8(2): 266. https://doi.org/10.3390/vaccines8020266.

Rees, E. E., Petukhova, T., Mascarenhas, M., Pelcat, Y., & Ogden, N. H. (2018). Environmental and social determinants of population vulnerability to Zika virus emergence at the local scale. *Parasites and Vectors*, *11*(1), 1–13. https://doi.org/10.1186/s13071-018-2867-8.

Tesla, B., Demakovsky, L. R., Mordecai, E. A., Ryan, S. J., Bonds, M. H., Ngonghala, C. N., Brindley, M. A., & Murdock, C. C. (2018). Temperature drives Zika virus transmission: Evidence from empirical and mathematical models. *Proceedings of the Royal Society B: Biological Sciences*, *285*(1884). https://doi.org/10.1098/rspb.2018.0795.

Yadav, S., Rawal, G., & Baxi, M. (2016). Zika virus: A pandemic in progress. *Journal of Translational Internal Medicine*, *4*(1), 42–45. https://doi.org/10.1515/jtim-2016-0009.

Index

A

Abiotic factors, 152, 158, 165
Aerosols, 10, 11, 55
Animal reservoirs, 6–8
Anthropogenic factors, 18, 151, 152
Antiviral medicines, 152
Arboviral, 18
Arboviruses, 152
Arenaviridae, 6, 144
Arthropods, 3, 152–154
Artificial intelligence, 12, 20, 37, 88
Artificial neural network, 24
Asymptomatic carrier, 25

B

Bacille Calmette-Guérin (BCG), 51
Bacillus thuringiensis, 121, 163
Biodiversity, 18, 19, 69, 70, 73, 74, 76
Biological treatment processes, 134
Bubonic plague, 85, 86

C

Chemotherapy, 48
Climatic factors, 83–86, 89–91
COVID-19, 2, 3, 5, 10, 18, 20–22, 25, 33–38, 41, 42, 48, 64, 65, 67, 68, 70–72, 75, 76, 119

D

Dengue, 18, 82, 88–91, 100–102, 104, 105, 152, 157, 163
Dengvaxia, 90, 105
Diesel exhaust particles (DEP), 57
Digitalisation, 75
DOTS, 52
Drug resistance, 52
Drug-resistant-strains (DR), 49

E

Ebola virus, 2, 6, 7, 19, 22, 64, 70
Ecological adaptation, 7
Economic outcomes, 42
Ectothermic, 86, 156
Electroencephalography (EEG), 91
El Niño, 18, 153, 159
Emerging pollutants, 118, 119, 126
Empirical relationships, 85
Encephalitis, 81–83, 90–92, 152
Endemic, 2, 12, 23, 51, 64, 67, 76, 134–136, 140, 143, 144, 154, 156, 164
Enteroviruses, 90
Environmental implications, 42
Environmental sustainability, 65
Enzyme-linked immunosorbent serologic assay (ELISA), 138
Epidemiology, 4, 5, 7, 9, 25, 135, 144
Epileptic seizures, 90–92
Ethambutol (ETH), 48

F

Flaviviridae, 6, 88, 100
Flaviviruses, 103, 105, 152, 156, 165
Fomites, 10, 11
Forecast modelling, 87
Fungal infections, 21

G

Global migration, 72
Global value chains, 34
Global warming, 18, 23, 35, 38, 40, 42, 49, 69, 71, 75, 82, 93, 102, 103, 157
Greenhouse gases, 18, 87
Gross domestic product (GDP), 34–36, 38, 40
Guillain–Barré syndrome, 100, 104, 105, 107, 108, 155

H

H5N1 (bird flu), 8, 9
Haemorrhagic fever, 6, 70, 134
Heat-shock protein, 19
HIV/AIDS, 2, 4–6, 33, 70
Host–pathogen interaction, 91
Host reservoirs, 160

I

Illegal wildlife trade, 75

Infectious diseases, 2, 18–21, 25, 64, 65, 67, 69, 72–76, 82, 87, 91, 102, 119
Influenza, 2, 3, 8, 9, 18–20, 22–23, 26, 55, 64, 65, 68, 70, 72, 155
Interferon-γ (IFN-γ), 51
Interleukin (IL)-1β, 51, 110
Intervention measures, 75
Isoniazid (INH), 48

J

Japanese encephalitis (JE), 91

L

Lassa fever, 2, 134–136, 138–145
Lassa virus, 134, 137, 138, 140
Lentivirus, 3

M

Machine learning, 88
Mastomys natalensis, 134–136, 144
Mathematical models, 157, 164
Membrane bioreactors, 118, 124, 126
Meteorological parameters, 92
Microcephaly, 99, 100, 105, 106, 109, 110, 155
Migration, 5, 7, 19, 24, 26, 57, 70, 84, 164, 165
Model-based prediction, 163
Mononegavirales, 6
Multi-faceted, 72, 75, 123
Multimammate rat, 134–136
Mycobacterium tuberculosis, 49, 164

N

Non-human primates, 3, 160, 163

O

One Health, 12, 25–26, 75

P

Parasitic helminths, 21
Personal protective equipment (PPE), 137
Phagosomes, 50
Polycyclic aromatic hydrocarbons (PAH), 56
Predictive modelling, 87
Primates, 3, 6, 160, 163

Q

Quarantined, 134, 140

R

Reactive nitrogen intermediates (RNIs), 50
Relative humidity, 22, 71, 86, 89, 91
Resilient species, 19
Retroviridae, 3
Reverse transcription-polymerase chain reaction (RT-PCR), 138
Rifampin (RIF), 48
Rift Valley fever, 18
RNA viruses, 3, 65, 152
Rodents, 3, 50, 85–87, 92, 136, 137, 139, 140

S

SARS-CoV, 2, 5, 9–11, 18, 67, 68
SARS-CoV-2, 5, 10, 11, 25, 48, 58, 68, 71
Serological, 101, 153, 165
Serotypes, 3, 88
Socio-economic factors, 7, 156, 158
Spanish flu, 2, 3, 8, 33, 64, 65, 67, 68
Streptomycin, 51, 52
Sub-Saharan Africa, 4, 5, 9, 12, 34, 35, 38, 134
Surveillance, 7, 9, 12, 52, 83, 92, 135, 141, 142, 153, 159, 164
surveillance systems, 52
Sylvatic spread, 161, 163

T

Tropical environments, 101
Tuberculosis, 47, 48
Tumour necrosis factor α (TNF-α), 51

V

Vaccination strategies, 75
Vector-borne, 12, 84, 91, 102, 155, 156
Viral transmission, 7, 154

W

Wolbachia bacterium, 90
Wolbachia pipientis, 163

Y

Yellow fever, 18, 88, 91, 101, 152, 153, 163
Yersinia pestis, 85–87

Z

ZIKV infections, 155, 156, 161, 163, 164
Zoonotic disease, 81–83, 85, 87, 89, 91, 92